Registered Health Information Administrator (RHIA) Exam Preparation

Tenth Edition

Patricia Shaw,
EdD, RHIA, FAHIMA

and

Darcy Carter,
DHSc, MHA, RHIA

Editors

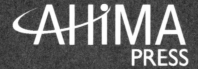

ISBN: 978-1-58426-928-1
eISBN: 978-1-58426-929-8

AHIMA Product No.: AB106023

AHIMA Staff:
Sarah Cybulski, MA, Assistant Editor
Megan Grennan, Director, Content Production and AHIMA Press
James Pinnick, Vice President, Content and Learning Solutions
Christine Scheid, Content Development Manager
Rachel Schratz, MA, Associate Digital Content Developer

Cover image: © 31moonlight31; iStock

**For more information, including updates, about AHIMA Press publications, visit
http://www.ahima.org/education/press.**

American Health Information Management Association
233 North Michigan Avenue, 21st Floor
Chicago, Illinois 60601-5809
ahima.org

Contents

About the Technical Editors

Patricia Shaw, EdD, RHIA, FAHIMA, holds a doctorate and master's degree in education. She is currently professor emeriti and adjunct professor at Weber State University, where she teaches quality and performance improvement, and coding courses. Prior to her position at Weber State, Dr. Shaw managed hospital health information management services departments and was a nosologist for 3M Health Information Systems. Dr. Shaw is also coauthor of *Quality and Performance Improvement in Healthcare: Theory, Practice, and Management* published by AHIMA.

Darcy Carter, DHSc, MHA, RHIA, earned her doctorate degree in health science with an emphasis in leadership and organizational behavior and her master's degree in healthcare administration. Dr. Carter is currently department chair, associate professor and MHA program director at Weber State University, where she teaches courses in coding, reimbursement, quality management, and healthcare management. Dr. Carter is also coauthor of *Quality and Performance Improvement in Healthcare: Theory, Practice, and Management* published by AHIMA.

Acknowledgments

AHIMA Press would like to thank Gretchen Jopp, MS, RHIA, CCS, CPC and Tamra K. Wood, RHIA, CCS, CCS-P, AHIMA Approved ICD-10-CM/PCS Trainer, for serving as technical reviewers of this edition.

About the RHIA Exam

Job opportunities for registered health information administrators (RHIAs) exist in multiple settings throughout the healthcare industry. These include the continuum of care delivery organizations, including hospitals, multispecialty clinics and physician practices, long-term care, mental health, and other ambulatory care settings. The profession has seen significant expansion in nonpatient care settings, with careers in managed care and insurance companies, software vendors, consulting services, government agencies, education, and pharmaceutical companies.

Working as a critical link between care providers, payers, and patients, an RHIA:

- Is an expert in managing patient health information and medical records, administering computer information systems, collecting and analyzing patient data, and using classification systems and medical terminologies.
- Possesses comprehensive knowledge of medical, administrative, ethical, and legal requirements and standards related to healthcare delivery and the privacy of protected patient information.
- Manages people and operational units, participates in administrative committees, and prepares budgets.
- Interacts with all levels of an organization—clinical, financial, administrative, and information systems—that employ patient data in decision-making and everyday operations.

The National Commission for Certifying Agencies (NCCA) has granted accreditation to AHIMA's RHIA certification program. This accomplishment establishes AHIMA as the industry leader in accredited health information and informatics management (HIIM) certification programs, and advances AHIMA's organizational mission of positioning AHIMA members and certificants as recognized leaders in advancing professional practice and standards in HIIM.

The Commission on Certification for Health Informatics and Information Management (CCHIIM) manages and sets the strategic direction for the certifications. Pearson Vue is the exclusive provider of AHIMA certification exams. To see sample questions and images of the new exam format, visit the AHIMA website.

Detailed information about the RHIA exam and academic eligibility requirements can be found at www.ahima.org/certification.

RHIA Exam Content Outline

Domain I: Data and Information Governance (17-20%)

- Evauate the integrity of the health record documentation
- Apply knowledge necessary to process the required clinical data elements for quality reporting (e.g., facility committees, payers)
- Understand and apply data dictionary standardization policies
- Manage documentation and data standards based on organizational policy
- Complete data analysis to inform management
- Develop policies and procedures for health record data, documentation management, and information governance
- Comply with retention and destruction policies for health information
- Manage the integrity of the master patient index (MPI)

Domain II: Compliance with Access, Use, and Disclosure of Health Information (15-18%)

- Manage patient access to their health information, including use of patient portals
- Advocate for patients and families in the process of obtaining health information
- Process health information requests according to legal and regulatory standards
- Monitor access to protected health information (PHI) internal and external to the organization (e.g., health information exchange [HIE])
- Develop health information request workflows to comply with legal and regulatory standards.
- Follow breach of information protocols.
- Ensure compliance with privacy and security initiatives (e.g., cyber security, disaster recovery)

Domain III: Data Analytics and Informatics (23-26%)

- Support end users in EHR applications
- Create reports and visual representations of data
- Use database management software and techniques (e.g., data mining)
- Audit documentation using a focused tool (e.g., clinical documentation integrity [CDI], quality, safety)
- Optimize health information and other technologies to improve workflows
- Support health information exchange [HIE] solutions
- Examine software applications and integrations for the impact to health information
- Validate healthcare statistics for organizational stakeholders
- Understand the information systems development life cycle, including the analysis, design/development, implementation, maintenance, and evaluation phases

Domain IV: Revenue Cycle Management (20-23%)

- Educate providers on various reimbursement models
- Validate coding accuracy
- Monitor Department of Health and Human Services (HHS) clinical documentation requirements
- Conduct clinical documentation integrity (CDI) activities in support of revenue and quality improvement initiatives
- Support the claims management process (e.g., CDM maintenance, DNFB analysis, and A/R management)
- Assign diagnoses and procedure codes and grouping according to official guidelines
- Conduct revenue integrity activities (e.g., coding audits, denials management, and fraud prevention)

Domain V: Management and Leadership (23-26%)

- Develop and implement goals and strategies, including change management to support organization initiatives
- Demonstrate knowledge of contracting/outsourcing processes
- Perform human resource management activities (e.g., recruiting staff, creating job descriptions, resolving personnel issues)
- Perform and oversee work design and process-improvement activities
- Facilitate training and development
- Prepare and implement budgets
- Assist with accreditation, licensing, or certification processes
- Monitor organizational compliance with health laws, regulations, or standards
- Demonstrate knowledge to lead or facilitate project management

How to Use This Book and Online Assessments

The RHIA practice questions and practice exams in this book and on the accompanying website test knowledge of content pertaining to the RHIA domains and tasks published by AHIMA and available at https://ahima.org/certification-careers/certification-exams/rhia/. The multiple-choice practice questions and examinations in this book and the accompanying website are presented in a similar format to those that might be found on the RHIA exam.

This book contains 520 multiple-choice questions and two multiple-choice practice exams (with 150 questions each). Because each question is identified with one of the 5 RHIA domains, you will be able to determine whether you need knowledge or skills in particular areas of the exam domains. Each question includes a rationale and reference with the correct answer. Pursuing the sources of these references will help you build your knowledge and skills in specific domains.

To use this book effectively, work through all of the practice questions first. This will help you identify areas in which you may need further preparation. For the questions that you answer incorrectly, read the associated references to help refresh your knowledge. After going through the practice questions, take one of the practice exams. Again, for the questions that you answer incorrectly, refresh your knowledge by reading the associated references. Continue in the same manner with the next practice exam.

Retake the practice questions and exams as many times as you like. Remember that to help build your knowledge and skills, you should review the references provided for all questions that you answered incorrectly.

The website presents the same RHIA practice questions and two timed practice exams printed in the book and also includes a bonus practice exam. (Practice Exam 3 is a web-only bonus exam.) These exams can be run in practice mode, which allows you to work at your own pace, or exam mode, which simulates the timed exam experience. The option to set the practice questions and simulated practice exams to be presented in random order exists, or you may choose to go through the questions in sequential order by domain. You may also choose to practice or test your skills on specific domains. For example, if you would like to build your skills in domain 2, you may choose only domain 2 questions for a given practice session.

Test-Taking Tips

The best way to prepare for the AHIMA RHIA Certification Exam is to study the material you have learned over the course of your health information administrator educational program. As it is difficult to remember everything you have learned over the course of the program, it is important to review the information. This is best done using this textbook and the tips found above in "How to Use This Book." Carefully review the information in the Commission on Certification for Health Informatics and Information Management Candidate Guide located in the accompanying website for this book (listed on the front, inside cover). You will want to prepare yourself mentally, physically, and emotionally to succeed.

Other tips while studying:

- Be sure to get enough sleep.
- Eat a healthy, well balanced diet.
- Stay hydrated.
- Take a break.
- Get some exercise.
- Do not try to memorize everything; work at understanding.
- Use tricks to remember the material, like using an acronym or other type of word or visual association.
- Try to eliminate other stressors, if possible.
- Take a practice exam in the three and one-half (3.5) hour time frame you will have for the exam.
- If you do not know where the testing center is located, visit it before the day of the exam. This will help you avoid getting lost or being late for your exam.
- Review the information on your Authorization to Test (ATT) letter.

Exam Day Tips

- Get enough sleep in the days leading up to the exam.
- Wear clothes that you are comfortable in and dress in layers so that you can remove or add a sweater based on the temperature of the room.
- Eat a good breakfast and give yourself enough time to get ready to leave so you are not rushed.
- Arrive at the testing center 30 minutes prior to your exam time with your required identification.
- You will have three and a half (3.5) hours to complete the exam. Do not obsess over the clock in the room, but do budget your time. This should allow you to answer each question and review any questions you may want to revisit. Time management will be an important part of taking the exam.
- Be sure to read each question carefully. Do not automatically assume you know the answer to a question without first reading the entire question and each answer choice carefully. After reviewing each answer, choose the best answer.
- Skip questions that you do not know the answer to or that are difficult and come back to them. You may find something in another question that helps you to recall information you need to answer a question you skipped. Be sure to manage your time well while you do this.
- Be sure to answer every test question. A "guess" is better than not taking the opportunity to answer a question. But, do so after carefully reviewing the question and the possible answers. After eliminating answers you know are incorrect, make the best selection. A true guess will give you a one-in-four chance of getting a question correct.
- Remember to relax as much as possible and BREATHE. You can do this!

PRACTICE QUESTIONS

Domain 1 *Data and Information Governance*

1. The HIM manager tasked the coding manager to development of a dashboard that shows the discharges pending final billing so that she can plan for staffing. Because this data changes throughout the day, what analysis technique is needed?

   a. Predictive modelling

   b. Indirect standardization

   c. Real-time analytics

   d. Data mining

2. A hospital employee destroyed a health record so that its contents—which would be damaging to the employee—could not be used at trial. In legal terms, the employee's action constitutes:

   a. Mutilation

   b. Destruction

   c. Spoliation

   d. Spoilage

3. The following descriptors about the data element DISCHARGE_DATE are included in a data dictionary: definition: date patient was discharged from the hospital; data type: date; field length: 15; required field: yes; default value: none; template: none. For this data element, data integrity would be better assured if:

   a. The template was defined

   b. The data type was numeric

   c. The field was not required

   d. The field length was longer

4. The HIM director at Community Hospital has noticed that history and physicals and operative reports are not being transcribed and returned by the transcription service within the negotiated timeframes. What should be her primary concern related to this issue?

   a. That the transcription service company will overcharge the hospital for reports that are delayed

   b. That physicians will stop dictating reports and just include comments in the progress notes

   c. That the Joint Commission will find that history and physicals are not being uploaded to the EHR system within the required 24-hour timeframe

   d. That information is not being made available in the patient portal within the required timeframe

5. Which statistics should a health data analyst recommend to a manager who would like to measure the relationship between length of stay and time to code a health record?

   a. Slope of the linear regression time

   b. T-test

   c. Correlation

   d. Intercept of the linear regression line

6. Danny, an HIM analyst for Memorial Hospital, is conducting a qualitative analysis of a discharged patient's chart. His goal in this process is:

   a. Determining if the documentation includes all requirements set by CMS, the state, and accrediting bodies

   b. Identifying whether all lab orders have corresponding lab reports in the chart

   c. Verifying that health professionals are providing appropriate care

   d. Ensuring the hospital bill is correct

7. Gladys was admitted to Sunshine Nursing Facility for rehabilitation following her hip fracture. Upon admission, the nursing staff assessed Gladys in multiple areas, some of which are cognitive loss, mood, vision function, pain, and the medications she is taking. This information will be recorded in her health record for the:

   a. Minimum data set to plan her care

   b. Pay-for-performance initiatives to manage payment

   c. Requirements of the CDC

   d. Identification of patients for NPSGs

8. In order to set the budget for next year, the hospital administrator tasked a business analyst with determining the average charges and average length of stay for Medicaid patients. The business analyst uses hospital claims data for this analysis and provides the results to the administrator. What type of data are the claims data in this case?

   a. Clinical data

   b. Statistical data

   c. Secondary data

   d. Primary data

9. The Western Hospital Corporation's HIM director wants to compare the time that each of the hospitals in the corporation are spending on chart analysis and determine how they are performing against the best practice standard. The HIM director generated the following data for comparison. What is this comparison process called?

Western Hospital Corporation				
HIM Corporate Dashboard				
April, 20xx				
	Analysis Days			Delinquency Rate
	IP	SDS	ED	
Community Region Facilities				
Hospital A	3.0	3.0	2.0	5%
Hospital B	1.0	2.0	1.0	0%
Hospital C	1.0	3.0	1.0	8%
Urban Region Facilities				
Hospital D	4.0	1.0	0.0	12%
Hospital E	2.0	32.0	30.0	23%
Hospital F	3.0	7.0	4.0	8%
Corporate Average	2.33	8.00	6.33	9%
Best Practice Standard	**2.0**	**2.0**	**1.0**	**<15%**

   a. Process comparison

   b. Outcome comparison

   c. Comparing

   d. Benchmarking

10. At Memorial Hospital, HIM professionals are located in the nursing stations, where they are responsible for all aspects of health record processing. While the patient is in the facility, the HIM professional does a daily concurrent review of the record. How does this assist the organization?

   a. By helping to remind providers to complete documentation requirements and sign orders, which is easier to do while the patient is still at the facility

   b. By indicating to physicians what documentation must be completed once the patient goes home

   c. By giving the billing department a list of all the charges to date for the patient

   d. By allowing the documentation to be uploaded to the patient portal for the patient to use after discharge

11. Hospitals often use master patient indexes to do which of the following?

   a. Analyze population-based data

   b. Determine survival rates

   c. Evaluate physicians

   d. Determine whether a patient has been seen in the facility before

12. Lisa, an HIM analyst for Healthwise Hospital, is conducting a quantitative analysis of a discharged patient's chart. Her goal in this process is:

    a. To ensure that the record is legible

    b. To identify deficiencies in the chart early so they can be corrected

    c. To verify that health professionals are providing appropriate care

    d. To ensure that the hospital bill is correct

13. Which of the following is the appropriate method for destroying electronic data?

    a. Burning

    b. Shredding

    c. Pulverizing

    d. Degaussing

14. John Smith, who was treated as a patient at a multihospital system, has three health record numbers. The term used to describe multiple health record numbers is:

    a. Unit record

    b. Overlay

    c. Overlap

    d. Integrity

15. What type of report would give administrators structured information in a variety of graphs to better plan facility operations?

    a. Enterprise master patient index

    b. Integrated delivery system

    c. Registration—admissions, discharge, transfer system

    d. Executive information system dashboard

16. Which of the following would *not* be an appropriate duty for an HIM professional?

    a. Documenting additions or deletions in a patient's record

    b. Monitoring documentation guidelines as set forth in legislation or regulatory standards

    c. Training care providers in documentation techniques

    d. Auditing patient records to determine the quality of the documentation

17. The insured party's member identification number is an example of which type of data?

    a. Demographic data

    b. Clinical data

    c. Certification data

    d. Financial data

18. A health data analyst has been asked to compile a report on the percentage of patients who had a baseline partial thromboplastin time (PTT) test performed prior to receiving heparin. What clinical reports in the health record would the health data analyst need to consult in order to prepare this report?

    a. Physician progress notes and medication record

    b. Nursing and physician progress notes

    c. Medication administration record and clinical laboratory reports

    d. Physician orders and clinical laboratory reports

19. City Hospital's revenue cycle management team has established the following benchmarks: (1) The value of discharged, not final billed (DNFB) cases should not exceed two days of average daily revenue; and (2) accounts receivable days are not to exceed 60 days. The net average daily revenue is $1,000,000. What do the following data indicate about how City Hospital is meeting its benchmarks?

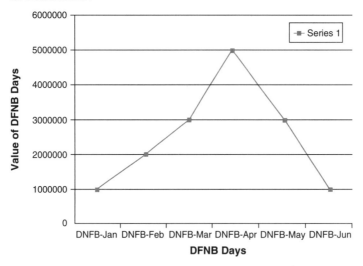

    a. DNFB cases met the benchmark 100 percent of the time.

    b. DNFB cases met the benchmark 75 percent of the time.

    c. DNFB cases met the benchmark 50 percent of the time.

    d. DNFB cases met the benchmark 25 percent of the time.

20. An analyst wishes to test the hypothesis that the wait time in the emergency department is longer on weekends than weekdays. What is the alternative hypothesis?

    a. The average wait time is shorter on weekends.

    b. The average wait time is longer on weekends.

    c. The average wait time is different on weekends and weekdays.

    d. The average wait time is the same on weekends and weekdays.

21. The data that describe other data in order to facilitate data quality are found in the:

    a. Data definition language

    b. Data dictionary

    c. Data standards

    d. Data definition

22. Bloodwork results from the laboratory information system, mammogram reports and films from the radiology information system, and a listing of chemotherapy agents administered to the patient from the pharmacy information system are all delivered into the patient's EHR. These different information systems that feed information into the EHR are known as:

    a. Interoperability

    b. Source systems

    c. Continuity of care records

    d. Clinical decision support systems

23. Which of the following processes is an ancillary function of the health record?

    a. Admitting and registration information

    b. Billing and reimbursement

    c. Patient assessment and care planning

    d. Biomedical research

24. While the focus of inpatient data collection is on the principal diagnosis, the focus of outpatient data collection is on the:

    a. Reason for admission

    b. Activities of daily living

    c. Discharge diagnosis

    d. Reason for encounter

25. The inpatient data set incorporated into federal law and required for Medicare reporting is the:

    a. Ambulatory Care Data Set

    b. Uniform Hospital Discharge Data Set

    c. Minimum Data Set for Long-term Care

    d. Health Plan Employer Data and Information Set

26. What is the main problem with using unstructured data for decision making?

    a. Cannot be stored in a database

    b. Lack of text-based processors

    c. Difficult to determine data completeness

    d. Takes more time to process the data

27. What document is a snapshot of a patient's status and includes everything from social issues to disease processes as well as critical paths and clinical pathways that focus on a specific disease process or pathway in a long-term care hospital (LTCH)?

    a. Face sheet

    b. Care plan

    c. Diagnosis plan

    d. Flow sheet

28. Which of the following personnel is authorized, per hospital policy, to take a physician's verbal order for the administration of medication?

    a. Unit secretary working on the unit where the patient is located

    b. Nurse working on the unit where the patient is located

    c. Health information director

    d. Admissions registrars

29. Name of element, definition, application in which the data element is found, locator key, ownership, entity relationships, date first entered system, date terminated from system, and system of origin are all examples of:

    a. Auto-authentication fields

    b. Metadata

    c. Data

    d. Information fields

30. Which statement is true about the following figure?

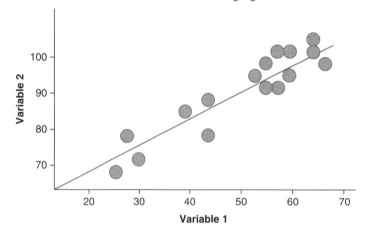

    a. There is no correlation between the variables.

    b. There is a negative relationship between the variables.

    c. There is a weak negative correlation between the variables.

    d. There is a positive relationship between the variables.

31. Which of the following represents dataflow for a hospital inpatient admission?

    a. Registration > diagnostic and procedure codes assigned > services performed > charges recorded

    b. Registration > services performed > charges recorded > diagnostic and procedure codes assigned

    c. Services performed > charges recorded > registration > diagnostic and procedure codes assigned

    d. Diagnostic and procedure codes assigned > registration > services performed > charges recorded

32. Which of the following is the goal of quantitative analysis performed by health information management (HIM) professionals?

    a. Ensuring the record is legible

    b. Identifying deficiencies early so they can be corrected

    c. Verifying that health professionals are providing appropriate care

    d. Checking to ensure bills are correct

33. To complete a comprehensive assessment and collect information for the Minimum Data Set for Long-Term Care, the coordinator must use which of the following?

    a. Core measure

    b. Resident Assessment Instrument

    c. Precertification

    d. Record of transfer

34. When managing the master patient index (MPI) which of the following would be the biggest concern for the health information professional?

    a. Physical space to house the server

    b. Number of computers in registration

    c. Maintaining the database

    d. Duplicate record numbers

35. How do healthcare providers use the administrative data they collect?

    a. For regulatory, operational, and financial purposes

    b. For statistical data purposes

    c. For electronic health record tracking purposes

    d. For continuity of patient care purposes

36. Data mapping is used to harmonize data sets or code sets. The code or data set from which the map originates is the:

    a. Source

    b. Target

    c. Equivalent group

    d. Solution

37. To ensure authentication of data entries, which type of signature is the most secure?

    a. Digital

    b. Electronic

    c. Handwritten

    d. Virtual

38. Mrs. Bolton is an angry patient who resents her physician "bossing her around." She refuses to take a portion of the medications the nurses bring to her pursuant to physician orders and is verbally abusive to the patient care assistants. Of the following options, the most appropriate way to document Mrs. Bolton's behavior in the patient health record is:

    a. Mean

    b. Noncompliant and hostile toward staff

    c. Belligerent and out of line

    d. A pain in the neck

39. Who is responsible for ensuring the quality of health record documentation?

    a. Board of directors

    b. Administrator

    c. Provider

    d. Health information management professional

40. A medical group practice has contracted with an HIM professional to help define the practice's legal health record. Which of the following should the HIM professional perform first to identify the components of the legal health record?

    a. Develop a list of all data elements referencing patients that are included in both paper and electronic systems of the practice

    b. Develop a list of statutes, regulations, rules, and guidelines that contain requirements affecting the release of health records

    c. Perform a quality check on all health record systems in the practice

    d. Develop a listing and categorize all information requests for health information over the past two years

41. According to the UHDDS definition, ethnicity should be recorded on a patient record as:

    a. Race of mother

    b. Race of father

    c. Hispanic, non-Hispanic

    d. Free-text descriptor as reported by patient

42. Which of the following is a component of the resident assessment instrument?

    a. The resident's health record

    b. A standard Minimum Data Set (MDS)

    c. Preadmission Screening Assessment

    d. Annual Resident Review

43. The EHR indicates that Dr. Anderson wrote the January 12 progress note at 11:04 a.m. We know Dr. Anderson wrote this progress note due to which of the following?

    a. Authorship

    b. Validation

    c. Integrity

    d. Identification

44. Which data set would be used to document an elective surgical procedure that does not require an overnight hospital stay?

    a. Uniform Hospital Discharge Data Set

    b. Data Elements for Emergency Department Systems

    c. Uniform Ambulatory Care Data Set

    d. Essential Medical Data Set

45. A coding supervisor audits coded records to ensure the codes reflect the actual documentation in the health record. This code auditing process addresses the data quality element of:

    a. Granularity

    b. Reliability

    c. Timeliness

    d. Accuracy

46. The purpose of the data dictionary is to _____ definitions and ensure consistency of use.

    a. Identify

    b. Standardize

    c. Create

    d. Organize

47. The process by which a person or entity who authored an EHR entry or document seeks to validate that they are responsible for the data contained within it is called:

    a. Endorsement

    b. Confirmation

    c. Authentication

    d. Consent

48. It is important for a healthcare entity to have _____ addressing how to deal with corrections made to erroneous entries in health records.

    a. Training sessions

    b. Policies and procedures

    c. Verbally communicated instructions

    d. A supervisory committee

49. A nurse tried to enter a temperature of 134 degrees and the system would not accept it. What is this an example of?

    a. Data collection

    b. Edit check

    c. Data reliability

    d. Hot spot

50. An alteration of the health information by modification, correction, addition, or deletion is known as a(n):

    a. Change

    b. Amendment

    c. Copy and paste

    d. Deletion

51. Keith is the supervisor of the MPI and chart deficiency review staff in the HIM department, which also includes being the liaison for the billing department and the R-ADT staff. He frequently meets with Michael, the R-ADT supervisor, to discuss methods to combat healthcare fraud and to verify that the patients are who they say they are and that they have the appropriate documentation for verification. This process is called:

    a. Consent management

    b. Identity management

    c. Identity matching

    d. Patient identification

52. The process of providing proof of the authorship of health record documentation is called:

    a. Identification

    b. Standardization of data capture

    c. Standardization of abbreviations

    d. Authentication

53. Which of the following plans address how information can be documented in the health record during down time or a catastrophic event?

    a. Disaster

    b. E-discovery response

    c. Business continuity

    d. Emergency documentation

54. The legal health record must meet requirements from the following:

    a. Federal regulations and AHIMA

    b. State laws and insurance companies

    c. State laws and accreditation body standards

    d. AHIMA and accreditation body standards

55. What is a legal document that is used to specify whether the patient would like to be kept on artificial life support if they become permanently unconscious or is otherwise dying and unable to speak for themselves?

    a. Durable power of attorney

    b. Living consent form

    c. Informed consent

    d. Advance directive

56. Records that are not completed by the physician within the time frame specified in the healthcare organization policies are called:

    a. Default records

    b. Delinquent records

    c. Loose records

    d. Suspended records

57. A patient born with a neural tube defect would be included in which type of registry?

    a. Birth defects

    b. Cancer

    c. Diabetes

    d. Trauma

58. Automated insertion of clinical data using templates or similar tools with predetermined components using uncontrolled and uncertain clinical relevance is an example of a potential breach of:

    a. Patient identification and demographic accuracy

    b. Authorship integrity

    c. Documentation integrity

    d. Auditing integrity

59. Records in disparate systems that do not communicate or do not have a logical relationship for record management are called:

    a. Electronic medical records

    b. Electronic health records

    c. Hybrid health records

    d. Computerized health records

60. An HIM professional designing a health record system for a healthcare entity should check _____ to find out how long health records should be retained by the entity.

    a. With the attending physician

    b. State and federal law

    c. County or city codes

    d. Joint Commission Accreditation Standards

61. The key to an effective retention and retrieval system of health records in a facility is:

    a. Master patient index

    b. Terminal digit filing

    c. Microfilm

    d. Optical imaging

62. The statement "All patients admitted with a diagnosis falling into ICD-10-CM code numbers S00 through T88" represents a possible case definition for what type of registry?

    a. Birth defect registry

    b. Cancer registry

    c. Diabetes registry

    d. Trauma registry

63. How long should the master patient index be maintained?

    a. For at least 5 years

    b. For at least 10 years

    c. For at least 25 years

    d. Permanently

64. Because a health record contains patient-specific data and information about a patient that has been documented by the professionals who provided care or services to that patient, it is considered:

    a. Secondary data source

    b. Aggregate data source

    c. Primary data source

    d. Reliable data source

65. The leadership and organizational structures, policies, procedures, technology, and controls that ensure that patient and other enterprise data and information sustain and extend the entity's mission and strategies, deliver value, comply with laws and regulations, minimize risk to all stakeholders, and advance the public good is called:

    a. Information asset management

    b. Information management

    c. Information governance

    d. Enterprise information management

66. Mary Smith, RHIA, has been charged with the responsibility of designing a data collection form to be used on admission of patients to the acute-care hospital in which she works. What is the first resource she should use?

    a. UHDDS

    b. UACDS

    c. MDS

    d. ORYX

67. Ensuring that only the most recent report is available for viewing is known as:

    a. Documentation integrity

    b. Authorship

    c. Validation

    d. Version control

68. In long-term care, the resident's comprehensive assessment is based on data collected in the:

    a. UHDDS

    b. OASIS

    c. MDS

    d. HEDIS

69. Which of the following are considered dimensions of data quality?

    a. Relevancy, granularity, timeliness, currency, accuracy, precision, and consistency

    b. Relevancy, granularity, timeliness, currency, atomic, precision, and consistency

    c. Relevancy, granularity, timeliness, concurrent, atomic, precision, and consistency

    d. Relevancy, granularity, equality, currency, precision, accuracy, and consistency

70. What is a primary purpose for documenting and maintaining health records?

    a. Effective communication among caregivers for continuity of care

    b. Substantiate claims for reimbursement

    c. Provide evidence for malpractice lawsuits

    d. Contribute to medical science

71. Which of the following is a retention concern with electronic health records?

    a. Durability

    b. Hardware obsolescence

    c. Storage space

    d. Statute of limitations

72. The practices or methods that defend against charges questioning the integrity of the data and documents are called:

    a. Authentication

    b. Security

    c. Accuracy

    d. Nonrepudiation

73. Which of the following indexes would be used to compare the number and quality of treatments for patients who underwent the same operation with different surgeons?

    a. Physician

    b. Master patient

    c. Procedure

    d. Disease and operation

74. Review of disease indexes, pathology reports, and radiation therapy reports is part of which function in the cancer registry?

    a. Case definition

    b. Case finding

    c. Follow-up

    d. Reporting

75. The medical staff at Regency Health is nationally renowned for its skill in performing cardiac procedures. The nursing staff in the cardiac unit has noticed that a significant number of health records do not have informed consents prior to the performance of procedures. Obtaining informed consent is the responsibility of the:

    a. Nursing staff

    b. Admissions department

    c. Physician

    d. Administration

76. A critical early step in designing an EHR in which the characteristics of each data element are defined is to develop a(n):

    a. Accreditation manual

    b. Core content

    c. Continuity of care record

    d. Data dictionary

77. Dr. Jones dies while still in active medical practice. He leaves incomplete records at Medical Center Hospital. The best way for the HIM department to handle these incomplete records is to:

    a. Have the administrator of the hospital complete them

    b. Have the charge nurse on the respective nursing units complete them

    c. Ask the chief of staff to complete them

    d. File the incomplete records with a notation about the physician's death

78. The first deliverable from a legal health record (LHR) definition project is a:

    a. List of LHR stakeholders

    b. Document matrix of LHR components

    c. Letter of support from management

    d. Master source system matrix

79. When data is taken from the health record and entered into registries and databases, the data in the registries or databases is then considered a(n):

    a. Secondary data source

    b. Reliable data source

    c. Primary data source

    d. Unreliable data source

80. The name of the government agency that has led the development of basic data sets for health records and computer databases is:

    a. The Centers for Medicare and Medicaid Services

    b. The National Committee on Vital and Health Statistics

    c. The American National Standards Institute

    d. The National Institute of Health

81. What term is used in reference to the systematic review of sample health records to determine whether documentation standards are being met?

    a. Qualitative analysis

    b. Legal record review

    c. Utilization analysis

    d. Ongoing record review

82. Which of the following is a concept designed to help standardize clinical content for sharing between providers?

    a. Continuity of care record

    b. Interoperability

    c. Personal health record

    d. SNOMED

83. A regular review of legal health record policies and procedures to ensure a healthcare entity remains in compliance with legal requirements is generally called a legal health record:

    a. Maintenance plan

    b. Management plan

    c. Attribute plan

    d. Strategic plan

84. Reviewing a health record for authentication and medical reports is called:

    a. Analysis

    b. Coding

    c. Assembly

    d. Indexing

85. Which of the following data sets would be most useful in developing a matrix for identification of components of the legal health record?

    a. Document name, media type, source system, electronic storage start date, stop printing start date

    b. Document name, media type

    c. Document name, medical record number, source system

    d. Document name, source system

86. This functionality can result in confusion from incessant repetition of irrelevant clinical data.

    a. Change

    b. Amendment

    c. Copy and paste

    d. Deletion

87. Personal information about patients such as their names, ages, and addresses is considered what type of information?

   a. Clinical

   b. Administrative

   c. Operational

   d. Accreditation

88. Bob Jones is considering contractors for his company's medical benefits, and he is reviewing health plans from two different entities. Which of the following databases should he consult to compare the performance of the two health plans?

   a. HEDIS

   b. OASIS

   c. ORYX

   d. UHDDS

89. In data quality management, the process of translating data into information to be utilized by an application is called:

   a. Analysis

   b. Warehousing

   c. Collection

   d. Application

90. Legally, which of the following is most important in determining the length of time a hospital must retain health records?

   a. Research needs

   b. Storage capabilities

   c. Statute of limitations

   d. Cost

91. Copies of personal health records (PHRs) are considered part of the legal health record when:

   a. Consulted by the provider to gain information on a consumer's health history

   b. Used by the healthcare entity to provide treatment

   c. Used by the provider to obtain information on a consumer's prescription history

   d. Used by the healthcare entity to determine a consumer's DNR status

92. Which information system is the gateway into a healthcare facility to identify if a patient has been treated there, contains demographic information to confirm patient identity, and shows if the patient has been treated at other facilities within an integrated delivery system (IDS)?

   a. HRIS

   b. EIS

   c. EMPI

   d. R-ADT

93. The Device and Media Controls Standard requires organizations to implement policies and procedures to:

    a. Address the final disposition of ePHI, hardware, and electronic media

    b. Restrict the types of media that can be used in the organization

    c. Restrict the type of hardware that can be used in the organization

    d. Address the hardware use for business associates

94. When a healthcare entity destroys health records after the acceptable retention period has been met, a certificate of destruction is created. How long must the healthcare entity maintain the certificate of destruction?

    a. 2 years

    b. 5 years

    c. 10 years

    d. Permanently

Domain 2 | *Compliance with Access, Use, and Disclosure of Health Information*

95. The legal health record for disclosure consists of:

   a. Any and all protected health information collected or used by a healthcare entity when delivering care

   b. Only the protected health information requested by an attorney for a legal proceeding

   c. The data, documents, reports, and information that comprise the formal business records of any healthcare entity that are to be utilized during legal proceedings

   d. All of the data and information included in the HIPAA designated record set

96. A secure method of communication between the healthcare provider and the patient is:

   a. Personal health record

   b. E-mail

   c. Patient portal

   d. Online health information

97. Based on which of the following concepts can a clinic requesting health records for one of its patients be reasonably assured that the correct patient information will be sent?

   a. Verification

   b. Confirmation

   c. Authentication

   d. Certification

98. In the state of California, healthcare organizations must provide patients a copy of their medical record within 15 days of the request, whereas HIPAA requires organizations to provide records within 30 days of the request. This is example of state law being _____ in relation to federal law.

   a. Stringent

   b. Contrary

   c. Standardized

   d. Conflicting

99. Recently, a healthcare organization has noticed an increase in the number of whooping cough cases in children under 5 years old. The healthcare organization reports the information to the state department of health. Which of the following statements is most applicable to the disclosure of this information?

   a. The healthcare organization violated HIPAA because it didn't get authorization prior to the disclosure.

   b. The healthcare organization did not violate HIPAA because it can disclose information to anyone as it sees fit.

   c. The healthcare organization did not violate HIPAA because the disclosure impacted the public health of everyone.

   d. The healthcare organization violated HIPAA because it did not get authorization from the state department of health prior to the disclosure.

100. The _____ requires organizations to implement policies and procedures to safeguard the facility and equipment from unauthorized access, tampering, and theft.

    a. Contingency plan

    b. Security Rule

    c. Media and device controls

    d. Emergency mode operations plan

101. Following a data breach with less than 500 impacted, how long does a covered entity have to provide notification of the breach to the secretary of the Department of Health and Human Services?

    a. Immediately after determination of the data breach

    b. Within 30 days

    c. Within 60 days

    d. 60 days after the end of the calendar year in which the breach occurred

102. Barbara requested a copy of her PHI from her physician office on August 31. It is now October 10 and she has not heard anything from the physician office. Which of the following statements is correct?

    a. This is not a HIPAA violation because the physician's office has 60 days to respond.

    b. This is not a HIPAA violation because Barbara does not have a right to her information.

    c. This is a HIPAA violation because the physician's office did not respond within 30 days.

    d. This is a HIPAA violation because the physician's office did not respond within 15 days.

103. Sara Anderson presented to the HIM department upset that her health information was sent to the state department of health. The HIM director explained to Sara that this information is part of their mandatory legal reporting requirements even though the information in her health record is owned by:

    a. The healthcare facility

    b. Sara's physician

    c. Sara, the patient

    d. The state

104. Gladys, a 90-year-old patient, calls the HIM department and tells the HIM professional that her daughter Joan will be in to pick up a copy of her records to take to her specialist. Which of the following is required for the HIM professional to comply with this request?

    a. Nothing is required; Gladys has provided her consent over the phone.

    b. Gladys must provide a written authorization.

    c. Gladys must repeat her request so that it can be verbally recorded.

    d. Joan must sign an authorization when she presents to the facility.

105. A physician is conducting a research study on the medication compliance of diabetic patients. The facility's consent-for-treatment form includes authorization for the use and disclosure of PHI for research, so the physician wants to begin the study. Why is this not acceptable?

    a. The Privacy Rule prohibits compound authorizations.

    b. Research does not require an authorization.

    c. The physician must call the participants of the study first.

    d. HIPAA prohibits the use and disclosure of information for research.

106. Mary Smith has gone to her doctor to discuss her current medical condition. What is the legal term that best describes the type of communication that has occurred between Mary and her physician?

    a. Closed communication

    b. Open communication

    c. Private communication

    d. Privileged communication

107. Community Hospital wants to provide transcription services for transcription of office notes of the private patients of physicians. All of these physicians have medical staff privileges at the hospital. This will provide an essential service to the physicians as well as provide additional revenue for the hospital. In preparing to launch this service, the HIM director is asked whether a business associate agreement is necessary. Which of the following should the hospital HIM director advise to comply with HIPAA regulations?

    a. Each physician practice should obtain a business associate agreement with the hospital.

    b. The hospital should obtain a business associate agreement with each physician practice.

    c. Because the physicians all have medical staff privileges, no business associate agreement is necessary.

    d. Because the physicians are part of an Organized Health Care Arrangement (OHCA) with the hospital, no business associate agreement is necessary.

108. Which of the following is a mechanism that records and examines activity in information systems?

    a. eSignature laws

    b. Security audits

    c. Minimum necessary rules

    d. Access controls

109. A patient requests copies of her medical records in an electronic format. The hospital maintains a portion of the designated record set in a paper format and a portion of the designated record set in an electronic format. How should the hospital respond?

    a. Provide the records in paper format only

    b. Scan the paper documents so that all records can be sent electronically

    c. Provide the patient with both paper and electronic copies of the record

    d. Inform the patient that PHI cannot be sent electronically

110. The HIM manager typically can testify about which of the following when a party in a legal proceeding is attempting to admit a health record as evidence?

    a. The care provided to the patient

    b. Identification of the record as the one subpoenaed

    c. The qualifications of the treating physician

    d. Identification of the standard of care used to treat the patient

111. If a healthcare provider is accused of breaching the privacy and confidentiality of a patient, what resource may a patient rely on to substantiate the provider's responsibility for keeping health information private?

    a. Professional Code of Ethics

    b. Federal Code of Fair Practice

    c. Federal Code of Silence

    d. State Code of Fair Practice

112. Which professional has the responsibility of determining when an individual or entity has the right to access healthcare information in a hospital setting?

    a. Physicians

    b. Nurses

    c. Health information management professionals

    d. Hospital administrators

113. Community Hospital is terminating its business associate relationship with a medical transcription company. The transcription company has no further need for any identifiable information that it may have obtained in the course of its business with the hospital. The CFO of the hospital believes that to be HIPAA compliant all that is necessary is for the termination to be in a formal letter signed by the CEO. In this case, how should the director of HIM advise the CFO?

    a. Confirm that a formal letter of termination meets HIPAA requirements and no further action is required

    b. Confirm that a formal letter of termination meets HIPAA requirements and no further action is required except that the termination notice needs to be retained for seven years

    c. Confirm that a formal letter of termination is required and that the transcription company must provide the hospital with a certification that all PHI that it had in its possession has been destroyed or returned

    d. Inform the CFO that business associate agreements cannot be terminated

114. Emma is getting ready to begin kindergarten. Her school is requesting her immunization records as required by state law. Per HIPAA, Emma's pediatrician may:

    a. Not disclose this PHI without the authorization of Emma's parent

    b. Disclose this information because it is not PHI

    c. Disclose this PHI with verbal permission from Emma's parent

    d. Not disclose this PHI because it is an exception to the public health activity authorization exception

115. Ensuring that data have been accessed or modified only by those authorized to do so is a function of:

    a. Data integrity

    b. Data quality

    c. Data granularity

    d. Logging functions

116. The privacy officer was conducting training for new employees and posed the following question to the trainees to help them understand the rule regarding breach notification: "If a breach occurs, which of the following must be provided to the individual whose PHI has been breached?"

    a. The facility's notice of privacy practices

    b. An authorization to release the individual's PHI

    c. The types of unsecured PHI that were involved

    d. A promise to never do it again

117. Community Hospital is planning implementation of various elements of the EHR in the next six months. Physicians have requested the ability to access the EHR from their offices and from home. What advice should the HIM director provide?

    a. HIPAA regulations do not allow this type of access.

    b. This access would be covered under the release of PHI for treatment purposes and poses no security or confidentiality threats.

    c. Access can be permitted providing that appropriate safeguards are put in place to protect against threats to security.

    d. Access cannot be permitted because the physicians would not be accessing information for treatment purposes.

118. The Medical Record Committee is reviewing the privacy policies for a large outpatient clinic. One of the members of the committee remarks that he feels that the clinic's practice of calling out a patient's full name in the waiting room is not in compliance with HIPAA regulations and that only the patient's first name should be used. Other committee members disagree with this assessment. What should the HIM director advise the committee?

    a. HIPAA does not allow a patient's name to be announced in a waiting room.

    b. There is no violation of HIPAA in announcing a patient's name, but the committee may want to consider implementing practices that might reduce this practice.

    c. HIPAA allows only the use of the patient's first name.

    d. HIPAA requires that patients be given numbers and that only the number be announced.

119. Which of the following is a kind of technology that focuses on data security?

    a. Clinical decision support

    b. Bitmapped data

    c. Firewalls

    d. Smart cards

120. Mr. Martin has asked his physician's office to review a copy of his PHI. His request must be responded to no later than _____ after the request was made.

    a. 90 days

    b. 60 days

    c. 30 days

    d. 6 weeks

121. A hospital currently includes the patient's social security number in the electronic version of the health record. The hospital risk manager has identified this as a potential identity breach risk and wants the information removed. The physicians and others in the hospital are not cooperating, saying they need the information for identification and other purposes. Given this situation, what should the HIM director suggest?

    a. Avoid displaying the number on any document, screen, or data collection field

    b. Allow the information in both electronic and paper forms since a variety of people need this data

    c. Require employees to sign confidentiality agreements if they have access to social security numbers

    d. Contact legal counsel for advice

122. The Privacy Rule establishes that a patient has the right of access to inspect and obtain a copy of his or her PHI:

    a. For as long as it is maintained

    b. For six years

    c. Forever

    d. For 12 months

123. Under the HIPAA Security Rule, these types of safeguards have to do with protecting the environment:

    a. Administrative

    b. Physical

    c. Security

    d. Technical

124. Which of the following is *not* an identifier under the Privacy Rule?

    a. Visa account 2773 985 0468

    b. Vehicle license plate BZ LITYR

    c. Age 75

    d. Street address 265 Cherry Valley Road

125. One of the four general requirements a covered entity must adhere to in order to be in compliance with the HIPAA Security Rule is to:

    a. Ensure the confidentiality, integrity, and addressability of ePHI

    b. Ensure the confidentiality, integrity, and accuracy of ePHI

    c. Ensure the confidentiality, integrity, and availability of ePHI

    d. Ensure the confidentiality, integrity, and accountability of ePHI

126. In Medical Center Hospital's clinical information system, nurses may write nursing notes and may read all parts of the patient health record for patients on the unit in which they work. This type of authorized use is called:

    a. Password limitation

    b. Security clearance

    c. Role-based access

    d. User grouping

127. Which of the following controls external access to a network?

    a. Access controls

    b. Alarms

    c. Encryption

    d. Firewall

128. Brittany is a new health information department employee. She is trained on the special procedures that must be followed prior to disclosure of health information that is deemed to be highly sensitive. Brittany knows that highly sensitive information receives special protections because it pertains to conditions that:

    a. Are generally fatal

    b. Are untreatable

    c. Are highly contagious

    d. Have a stigma or sensitivity associated with them

129. If a patient has health insurance but pays in full for a healthcare service and asks that the information be kept private, under HIPAA the covered entity must:

    a. Release the information to the health insurance provider

    b. Get special patient consent to release the information

    c. Comply with the patient's request and keep the information private

    d. Request permission from HHS to release the information

130. Identifying appropriate users of specific information is a function of:

    a. Access control

    b. Nosology

    c. Data modeling

    d. Workflow modeling

131. A visitor sign-in sheet to a computer area is an example of what type of control?

    a. Administrative

    b. Audit

    c. Facility access

    d. Workstation

132. Which of the following is an administrative safeguard action?

    a. Facility access control

    b. Documentation retention guidelines

    c. Maintenance record

    d. Media reuse

133. Susan is completing her required high school community service hours by serving as a volunteer at the local hospital. Relative to the hospital, Susan is a(n):

    a. Business associate

    b. Employee

    c. Workforce member

    d. Covered entity

134. What is the legal term used to define the protection of health information in a patient–provider relationship?

    a. Access

    b. Confidentiality

    c. Privacy

    d. Security

135. Mary Jones has been declared legally incompetent by the court. Mrs. Jones's sister has been appointed her legal guardian. Her sister requested a copy of Mrs. Jones's health records. Of the options listed here, what is the best course of action?

    a. Comply with the sister's request but first request documentation from the sister that she is Mary Jones's legal guardian

    b. Provide the information as requested by the sister

    c. Require that Mary Jones authorize the release of her health information to the sister

    d. Refer the sister to Mary Jones's doctor

136. Caitlin has been experiencing abdominal pain. Removal of her gallbladder was recommended. Who is responsible to obtain Caitlin's informed consent?

    a. The anesthesiologist who will be administering general anesthesia

    b. The surgical nurse who will assist during surgery

    c. The physician who will be performing the surgery

    d. The administrator in the surgery department

137. Health Insurance Portability and Accountability Act's Privacy Rule states that "_____ used for the purposes of treatment, payment, or healthcare operations does not require patient authorization to allow providers access, use, or disclosure." However, only the _____ information needed to satisfy the specified purpose can be used or disclosed.

    a. Demographic information, minimum necessary

    b. Protected health information, minimum necessary

    c. Protected health information, diagnostic

    d. Demographic information, diagnostic

138. The HIM manager received notification that a user accessed the PHI of a patient with the same last name as the user. This is an example of a(n):

    a. Encryption

    b. Trigger flag

    c. Transmission security

    d. Redundancy

139. Which of the following is a direct command that requires an individual or a representative of a healthcare entity to appear in court or to present an object to the court?

    a. Judicial decision

    b. Subpoena

    c. Credential

    d. Regulation

140. Kay Denton wrote to Mercy Hospital requesting an amendment to her PHI. She states that her record incorrectly lists her weight at 180 lbs. instead of her actual 150 lbs., and amending it would look better on her record. The information is present on a copy of a history and physical that General Hospital sent to Mercy Hospital. Mercy Hospital may decline to grant her request based on which privacy rule provision?

    a. Individuals do not have the right to make amendment requests.

    b. The history and physical was not created by Mercy Hospital.

    c. A history and physical is not part of the designated record set.

    d. Mercy Hospital must grant her request.

141. Authorization management involves:

    a. The process used to protect the reliability of a database

    b. Limiting user access to a database

    c. Allowing unlimited use of the database

    d. Developing definitions for database elements

142. Per HITECH, an accounting of disclosures must include disclosures made during the previous:

    a. 10 years

    b. 6 years

    c. 3 years

    d. 1 year

143. In the case of behavioral healthcare information, a healthcare provider may disclose health information on a patient without the patient's authorization in which of the following situations?

    a. Court order, duty to warn, and involuntary commitment proceedings

    b. Duty to warn, release of psychotherapy notes, and court order

    c. Involuntary commitment proceedings, court order, and substance abuse treatment records

    d. Release of psychotherapy notes, substance abuse treatment records, and duty to warn

144. An employee received an email that he thought was from the information technology department. He provided his personal information at the sender's request. The employee was tricked by:

    a. Phishing

    b. Ransomware

    c. Virus

    d. Bot

145. City Hospital has implemented a procedure that allows inpatients to decide whether they want to be listed in the hospital's directory. The directory information includes the patient's name, location in the hospital, and general condition. If a patient elects to be in the directory, this information is used to inform callers who know the patient's name. Some patients have requested that they be listed in the directory, but information is to be released to only a list of specific people the patient provides. A hospital committee is considering changing the policy to accommodate these types of patients. In this case, what type of advice should the HIM director provide?

    a. Approve the requests because this is a patient right under HIPAA regulations

    b. Deny these requests because screening of calls is difficult to manage and if information is given in error, this would be considered a violation of HIPAA

    c. Develop two different types of directories—one directory for provision of all information and one directory for provision of information to selected friends and family of the patient

    d. Deny these requests and seek approval from the Office of Civil Rights

146. A competent adult female has a diagnosis of ovarian cancer and while on the operating table suffers a stroke and is in a coma. Her son would like to access her health records from a clinic she recently visited for pain in her right arm. The patient is married and lives with her husband and two grown children. According to the Uniform Health Care Decisions Act (UHCDA), who is the logical person to request and sign an authorization to access the woman's health records from the clinic?

    a. Adult child making request

    b. Oldest adult child

    c. Patient

    d. Spouse

147. The baby of a mother who is 15 years old was recently discharged from the hospital. The mother is seeking access to the baby's health record. Who must sign the authorization for release of the baby's health record?

    a. Both mother and father of the baby

    b. Maternal grandfather of the baby

    c. Maternal grandmother of the baby

    d. Mother of the baby

148. The outpatient clinic of a large hospital is reviewing its patient sign-in procedures. The registration clerks say it is essential that they know if the patient has health insurance and the reason for the patient's visit. The clerks maintain that having this information on a sign-in sheet will make their jobs more efficient and reduce patient waiting time in the waiting room. What should the HIM director advise in this case?

   a. To be HIPAA compliant, sign-in sheets should contain the minimal information necessary such as patient name.

   b. Patient name, insurance status, and diagnoses are permitted by HIPAA.

   c. Patient name, insurance status, and reason for visit would be considered incidental disclosures if another patient saw this information.

   d. Any communication overheard by another patient is considered an incidental disclosure.

149. The Latin phrase meaning "let the master answer" that puts responsibility for negligent actions of employees on the employer is called:

   a. *Res ipsa locquitor*

   b. *Res judicata*

   c. *Respondeat superior*

   d. *Restitutio in integrum*

150. Employees in the hospital business office may have legitimate access to patient health information without patient authorization based on what HIPAA standard or principle?

   a. Minimum necessary

   b. Compound authorization

   c. Accounting of disclosures

   d. Preemption

151. Per the HITECH breach notification requirements, which of the following is the threshold in which the media and the Secretary of Health and Human Services should be notified of the breach?

   a. more than 1,000 individuals affected

   b. more than 500 individuals affected

   c. more than 250 individuals affected

   d. Any number of individuals affected requires notification

152. Dr. Williams is on the medical staff of Sutter Hospital, and he has asked to see the health record of his wife, who was recently hospitalized. Dr. Jones was the patient's physician. Of the options listed here, which is the best course of action?

   a. Refer Dr. Williams to Dr. Jones and release the record if Dr. Jones agrees

   b. Inform Dr. Williams that he cannot access his wife's health information unless she authorizes access through a written release of information

   c. Request that Dr. Williams ask the hospital administrator for approval to access his wife's record

   d. Inform Dr. Williams that he may review his wife's health record in the presence of the privacy officer

153. Which of the following are technologies and methodologies for rendering protected health information unusable, unreadable, or indecipherable to unauthorized individuals as a method to prevent a breach of PHI?

    a. Encryption and destruction

    b. Recovery and encryption

    c. Destruction and redundancy

    d. Interoperability and recovery

154. The hospital's public relations department in conjunction with the local high school is holding a job shadowing day. The purpose of this event is to allow high school seniors an opportunity to observe the various jobs in the hospital and to help the students with career planning. The public relations department asks for input on this event from the standpoint of HIPAA compliance. In this case, what should the HIM department advise?

    a. Job shadowing is allowed by HIPAA under the provision of allowing students and trainees to practice.

    b. Job shadowing should be limited to areas in which the likelihood of exposure to PHI is very limited, such as administrative areas.

    c. Job shadowing is allowed by HIPAA under the provision of volunteers.

    d. Job shadowing is specifically prohibited by HIPAA.

155. A hospital releases information to an insurance company with proper authorization by the patient. The insurance company forwards the information to a medical data clearinghouse. This process is referred to as:

    a. Admissibility

    b. Civil release

    c. Privileging process

    d. Redisclosure

156. When a patient revokes authorization for release of information after a healthcare entity has already released the information, the healthcare entity in this case:

    a. May be prosecuted for invasion of privacy

    b. Has become subject to civil action

    c. Has violated the security regulations of HIPAA

    d. Is protected by the Privacy Act

157. Generally, policies addressing the confidentiality of quality improvement (QI) committee data (minutes, actions, and so forth) state that this kind of data is:

    a. Protected from disclosure

    b. Subject to release with patient authorization

    c. Generally available to interested parties

    d. May not be reviewed or released to external reviewers such as the Joint Commission

158. An employer has contacted the HIM department and requested health information on one of his employees. Of the options listed here, what is the best course of action?

    a. Provide the information requested

    b. Refer the request to the attending physician

    c. Request the employee's written authorization for release of information

    d. Request the employer's written authorization for release of the employee's information

159. Under the HIPAA Privacy Rule, a hospital may disclose health information without authorization or subpoena in which of the following cases?

    a. The patient has been involved in a crime that may result in death.

    b. The patient has celebrity status and requires protection.

    c. The father of a 22-year-old is requesting the records.

    d. An attorney requests records.

160. Covered entities must retain documentation of their security policies for at least:

    a. Five years

    b. Five years from the date of origination

    c. Six years from the date when last in effect

    d. Six years from the date of the last incident

161. Under HIPAA, when is the patient's written authorization required to release his or her healthcare information?

    a. For purposes related to treatment

    b. For purposes related to payment

    c. For administrative healthcare operations

    d. For any purpose unrelated to treatment, payment, or healthcare operations

162. Notices of privacy practices must be available at the site where the individual is treated and:

    a. Must be posted next to the entrance

    b. Must be posted in a prominent place where it is reasonable to expect that patients will read them

    c. May be posted anywhere at the site

    d. Do not have to be posted at the site

163. The HIM director has been asked to secure the record of patient John Smith due to impending ligation in a legal hold. The concept of legal hold requires:

    a. Special, tracked handling of patient records involved in litigation to ensure no changes can be made

    b. Attorneys for healthcare entities to stop all activity with records involved in litigation

    c. All records involved in litigation to be printed and held in a locked cabinet

    d. To not allow further documentation to occur in any record involved in litigation

164. Regarding an individual's right of access to their own PHI, per HIPAA, a covered entity:

    a. Must act on the request within 90 days

    b. May extend its response by 60 days if it gives the reasons for the delay

    c. May require individuals to make their requests in writing

    d. Does not have limits regarding what it can charge individuals for copies of their health records

165. Central City Clinic has requested that Ghent Hospital send its hospital records from Susan Hall's most recent admission to the clinic for her follow-up appointment. Which of the following statements is true?

    a. The Privacy Rule requires that Susan Hall complete a written authorization.

    b. The hospital may send only discharge summary, history, and physical and operative report.

    c. The Privacy Rule's minimum necessary requirement does not apply.

    d. This "public interest and benefit" disclosure does not require the patient's authorization.

166. A federal confidentiality statute specifically addresses confidentiality of health information about _____ patients.

    a. Developmentally disabled

    b. Elderly

    c. Drug and alcohol recovery

    d. Cancer

167. The confidentiality of incident reports is generally protected in cases when the report is filed in:

    a. The nursing notes

    b. The patient's health record

    c. The physician's progress notes

    d. The hospital risk manager's office

168. Which one of the following has access to personally identifiable data without authorization or subpoena?

    a. Law enforcement in a criminal case

    b. The patient's attorney

    c. Public health departments for disease reporting purposes

    d. Workers' compensation for disability claim settlement

169. An original goal of HIPAA Administrative Simplification was to standardize:

    a. Privacy notices given to patients

    b. The electronic transmission of health data

    c. Disclosure of information for treatment purposes

    d. The definition of PHI

170. The privacy officer was conducting training for new employees and posed the following question to the trainees to help them understand the rule regarding protected health information (PHI): "Which of the following is an element that makes information 'PHI' under the HIPAA Privacy Rule?"

    a. Identifies an attending physician

    b. Specifies the insurance provider for the patient

    c. Contained within a personnel file

    d. Relates to one's health condition

171. A nurse administrator who is not typically on call to cover staffing shortages gets called in over the weekend to staff the emergency department. She does not have access to enter notes since this is not a part of her typical role. In order to meet the intent of the HIPAA Security Rule, the hospital policy should include a:

    a. Requirement for her to attend training before accessing ePHI

    b. Provision for another nurse to share his or her password with the nurse administrator

    c. Provision to allow her emergency access to the system

    d. Restriction on her ability to access ePHI

172. The Breach Notification Rule requires covered entities to establish a process for investigating whether a breach has occurred and which of the following?

    a. Establish a new position for a Privacy Officer

    b. Notify affected individuals when a breach occurs

    c. Establish a policy on minimum necessary

    d. Notify the primary care physicians of all patients of the breach

173. Which of the following is considered a two-factor authentication system?

    a. User ID and password

    b. User ID and voice scan

    c. Password and swipe card

    d. Password and PIN

174. Which of the following is a "public interest and benefit" exception to the authorization requirement?

    a. Payment

    b. PHI regarding victims of domestic violence

    c. Information requested by a patient's attorney

    d. Treatment

175. Which of the following statements is true in regard to training in protected health information (PHI) policies and procedures?

    a. Every member of the covered entity's workforce must be trained.

    b. Only individuals employed by the covered entity must be trained.

    c. Training only needs to occur when there are material changes to the policies and procedures.

    d. Documentation of training is not required.

176. Under the Privacy Rule, which of the following must be included in a patient accounting of disclosures?

    a. State-mandated report of a sexually transmitted disease

    b. Disclosure pursuant to a patient's signed authorization

    c. Disclosure necessary to meet national security or intelligence requirements

    d. Disclosure for payment purposes

Domain 3 *Data Analytics and Informatics*

177. A computer software program that supports a coder in assigning correct codes is called a(n):

    a. Encoder

    b. Grouper

    c. Automated coder

    d. Decision support system

178. A coding service had 400 discharged accounts to code in March. The service coded 200 within 3 days, 100 within 5 days, 50 within 8 days, and 50 within 10 days. The average turnaround time for coding in March was:

    a. 3 days

    b. 5 days

    c. 6.5 days

    d. 9 days

179. An organization's productivity standards should reflect its:

    a. Goals

    b. Vision

    c. Procedures

    d. Affinity groupings

180. The fact that a patient entered data into an EHR via a portal is:

    a. Administrative metadata

    b. Captured in a data model

    c. E-discovery

    d. Software programming

181. A physician on your staff asked you to help her collect information about the effects of smoking during pregnancy on the birth weight of babies. You were asked to collect the following information: whether or not the mothers smoke during pregnancy; birth weight of the babies; Apgar scores at one minute; and Apgar scores at five minutes. The scales of these variables would be:

    a. Nominal, ordinal, interval, ratio

    b. Nominal, ratio, ordinal, ordinal

    c. Ordinal, nominal, ratio, interval

    d. Ratio, ordinal, interval, nominal

182. The root cause of poor quality of data in the EHR can be determined by:

    a. Benchmarking against best practices

    b. Determining patient mortality rates

    c. Measuring patient care outcomes

    d. Observing how an EHR is used

183. Which statistical inference measures both the strength of a relationship between two variables and the functional relationship between them?

   a. Correlation

   b. T-test

   c. Simple linear regression

   d. Standard deviation

184. In which phase of the modern systems development life cycle does determining the budget, schedule, and personnel constraints occur?

   a. Monitoring of results

   b. Identification of need

   c. Maintenance

   d. Implementation

185. Which of the following is a task performed during system customization?

   a. Adjusting decision support rules

   b. Data conversion

   c. Testing

   d. Workflow and process improvement

186. An example of EHR data stewardship that would be required of the average healthcare professional is:

   a. Contributing to the design and development of data requirements for an EHR

   b. Ensuring that structured data is entered when such a choice is available in an EHR

   c. Maintaining EHR data in an appropriately configured information system

   d. Not sharing EHR data with others who have a need to know

187. The establishment of a shared set of behaviors and standards that enable health information exchange among a HIE's participants is called:

   a. Governance

   b. Trust community

   c. Workflows

   d. Interoperability standards

188. In order to effectively transmit healthcare data between a provider and a payer, both parties must adhere to which electronic data interchange standards?

   a. DICOM

   b. IEEE 1073

   c. LOINC

   d. ASC X12

189. The surgery department is evaluating its postoperative infection rate of 6 percent. The chief of surgery asks the quality improvement coordinator to find the postoperative infection rates of 10 similar hospitals in the same geographic region to see how the rates compare. This process is called:

    a. Benchmarking

    b. Critical pathway analysis

    c. Internal comparisons

    d. Universal precautions

190. Identify the level in the data model that describes how the data is stored within the database:

    a. Conceptual data model

    b. Physical data model

    c. Logical data model

    d. Data manipulation language

191. To ensure quality of data, the cancer committee reviews the abstracting done by the cancer registry personnel. This type of reliability check is called:

    a. Precision

    b. Recheck

    c. Interrater

    d. Construct

192. Which work measurement tool uses random sample observations to obtain information about the performance of an entire department?

    a. Performance measurement

    b. Work distribution

    c. Work sampling

    d. Performance controls

193. In addition to bar codes on health record documents, what other forms of recognition characteristics enhance the accuracy of form indexing features?

    a. Access controls

    b. COLD

    c. OCR

    d. Workflow

194. A hospital allows their coding professionals to work at home. The hospital is in the process of identifying strategies to minimize the security risks associated with this practice. Which of the following would be best to ensure that data breaches are minimized when the home computer is unattended?

    a. User name and password

    b. Automatic session terminations

    c. Cable locks

    d. Encryption

195. Which of the following statements is true of structured query language (SQL)?

    a. It is both a data manipulation and data back-up mechanism.

    b. It defines data elements and manipulates and controls data.

    c. It is the computer language associated with document imaging.

    d. Users are not able to query a relational database.

196. In which of the following processes does an analyst perform exploratory data analysis to determine trends and identify patterns in the data set?

    a. Data quality

    b. Data mining

    c. Record analysis

    d. Inferential statistics

197. A radiology department is planning to develop a remote clinic and transmit images for diagnostic purposes. The most important set of standards to implement for image transmission is:

    a. X12N

    b. LOINC

    c. IEEE 1073

    d. DICOM

198. Protocols that support communication between applications are often referred to as:

    a. Application program

    b. Interface code

    c. Messaging standards

    d. Source code

199. Which graph is the best choice when exploring the relationship between length of stay and charge for a set of patients?

    a. Line graph

    b. Bar chart

    c. Pie chart

    d. Scatter diagram

200. A single point of personalized web access through which to find and deliver information, applications, and services is called a(n):

    a. Keyhole

    b. Entry way

    c. WWW

    d. Portal

201. The process of integrating healthcare facility systems requires the creation of:

    a. Data warehouses

    b. E-health initiatives

    c. Enterprise master patient indexes

    d. Electronic data interchange

202. The performance standard "Transcribe 1,500 lines per day" is an example of a:

    a. Quality standard

    b. Quantity standard

    c. Joint Commission standard

    d. Compliance standard

203. For an EHR to provide robust clinical decision support, what critical element must be present?

    a. Structured data

    b. Internet connection

    c. Physician portal

    d. Standard vocabulary

204. The computer abstracting system in a facility has an edit that does not allow coders to assign obstetrical codes to male patients. This edit is called a(n):

    a. Preventive control

    b. Feedback control

    c. Performance measure

    d. Audit trail

205. Community Hospital just added a new system that changed the way data move throughout the facility. Which of the following would need to be updated to reflect this change?

    a. Data dictionary

    b. Entity relationship diagram

    c. Dataflow diagram

    d. Semantic object model

206. The benefits patients experience when using a patient portal include all of the following *except* being able to:

    a. Edit their medical record information

    b. View lab results

    c. Update demographics

    d. Send messages to their providers

207. This type of data display tool is used to show the relationship of each part to the whole.

    a. Pie charts

    b. Bar graphs

    c. Line graphs

    d. Histogram

208. When is the best time to map current processes?

    a. During the EHR planning stageJ

    b. In the process of selecting the vendor

    c. While implementation is occurring

    d. After go-live

209. A quality coding review that is based on specific problems identified during an initial baseline review in a hospital is called a(n):

    a. Focused coding review

    b. Compliance initiative

    c. Internal audit

    d. Concurrent review

210. Which of the following is the goal of an MPI ongoing maintenance program?

    a. To maintain low creation rates for duplicates, overlaps, and overlays

    b. To maintain the readmission rate for the facility

    c. To carry out treatment, payment, and operations

    d. To ensure appropriate state regulations of insurance and health plans

211. Which model for health information exchange stores patient records in a single database built to allow queries into the system?

    a. Federated

    b. Hybrid

    c. Centralized

    d. Decentralized

212. Which of the following is an organization that develops standards related to the interoperability of health information technology?

    a. National Health Information Network

    b. National Committee on Vital and Health Statistics

    c. Health Level 7

    d. EHR Collaborative

213. A network made accessible to trusted individuals outside of the facility is called a(n):

    a. Extranet

    b. Intranet

    c. VPN

    d. LAN

214. When performing an internal audit for coding compliance, which of the following would be suitable case selections for auditing?

    a. Infrequent diagnosis and procedure codes

    b. Medical and surgical MS-DRGs by low dollar and low volume

    c. Medical and surgical MS-DRGs by high dollar and high volume

    d. Low-volume admission diagnoses

215. An analyst wishes to use the CMI for a set of MS-DRGs to determine if a documentation improvement program is having an impact. Use the MS-DRG volumes and weights in the following table to calculate the CMI for the three MS-DRGs.

MS-DRG	Description	Weight	Volume
034	CAROTID ARTERY STENT PROCEDURE W MCC	3.9994	100
035	CAROTID ARTERY STENT PROCEDURE W CC	2.2838	52
036	CAROTID ARTERY STENT PROCEDURE W/O CC/MCC	1.8807	36

    a. 2.2838

    b. 3.1192

    c. 3.9994

    d. 3.2345

216. Which of the following represents the correct sequence (from low to high) of levels of interoperability?

    a. Semantic, basic, functional

    b. Basic, functional, semantic

    c. Functional, process, semantic

    d. Functional, semantic, basic

217. You want to graph the average length of stay by sex and service for the month of April. Which graphic tool would you use?

    a. Bar graph

    b. Histogram

    c. Line graph

    d. Pie chart

218. A requirements specification that lists what is needed from the vendor to support interoperability is necessary to:

    a. Create a checklist of user concerns about information systems

    b. Identify specific features and functions that must be in an information system

    c. Make a migration path for future phases of information systems

    d. Verify that an information system works as anticipated

219. The distinguishing feature of a results management application is that it:

    a. Captures charges for diagnostic studies and sends them to a billing system

    b. Directs the work of the departments that produce results of diagnostic studies

    c. Enables results of a diagnostic study to be compared and displayed with other data

    d. Provides diagnostic study information in viewable form

220. If an analyst wishes to determine the root cause of claim denials during June via a random sample, what is the sampling unit?

    a. Patient

    b. Hospital

    c. Claim

    d. Payer

221. Which of the following is an example of demographic data?

    a. 125 Oak Street, Smallville, KS

    b. Mother died of heart disease

    c. Temperature: 100 degrees F

    d. History of appendectomy at age 4

222. Once a current process is mapped, the next step should be:

    a. Assess for improvement

    b. Compare against EHR capabilities

    c. Develop new policies and procedures

    d. Validate completeness and accuracy

223. A signed patient consent form scanned into an EHR is an example of:

    a. Discrete data

    b. Image data

    c. Narrative data

    d. Structured data

224. In which phase of the modern systems development life cycle does negotiating the contract occur?

    a. Acquisition

    b. Specification of requirements

    c. Maintenance

    d. Monitoring of results

225. A clinic that is expanding its service offerings and needs an individual to help design a new database will be searching for a:

    a. Data administrator

    b. Database administrator

    c. Data governance manager

    d. Data technologist

226. A researcher mined the Medicare Provider Analysis Review (MEDPAR) file. The analysis revealed trends in lengths of stay for rural hospitals. What type of investigation was the researcher conducting?

   a. Content analysis

   b. Effect size review

   c. Psychometric assay

   d. Secondary analysis

227. A data model is used to:

   a. Define every data element in an information system

   b. Describe how data are used in creating information

   c. Display information to users in a meaningful way

   d. List the attributes of data

228. A way to assess the quality of data in the EHR is to:

   a. Audit structured data entries

   b. Compare data in the EHR to dictated documents

   c. Determine an acceptable error rate

   d. Review data against established norms

229. A healthcare facility has decided to adopt a tool that helps with multidisciplinary care planning. What tool meets these criteria?

   a. Clinical pathways

   b. Clinical practice guidelines

   c. Clinical provider order entry

   d. Electronic health record

230. Which of the following statements justifies the use of a dashboard?

   a. It facilitates budget development.

   b. It manages information system projects.

   c. It utilizes statistical techniques.

   d. It monitors key measures.

231. The performance standard "Complete five birth certificates per hour" is an example of a:

   a. Quality standard

   b. Quantity standard

   c. Joint Commission standard

   d. Compliance standard

232. This type of chart is used to focus attention on any variation in a process and helps the team to determine whether that variation is normal or a result of special circumstances.

    a. Pareto chart

    b. Pie chart

    c. Control chart

    d. Line chart

233. The decision has been made to perform data mining to determine where the skilled nursing facility is profitable and where there is a loss. Identify a data mining technique that could be used.

    a. Association rule learning

    b. Normalization

    c. Computer-aided software engineering

    d. Data modeling

234. You have been asked by the Chief Medical Officer of ABC Hospital to do research on the COVID-19 pandemic in your community and its impact on the hospital. You start out with determining the average age, median length of stay, gender and race admission rates, and insurance coverage. Identify the type of data analytics performed in this scenario.

    a. descriptive analytics

    b. diagnostic analytics

    c. predictive analytics

    d. prescriptive analytics

235. What type of interoperability addresses the medical words, phrases, and terms used in healthcare and their definitions so that there is clear and consistent usage among all EHR systems?

    a. Process

    b. Technical

    c. Semantic

    d. Syntactic

236. What component of an EHR provides communication between clinical and administrative staff members, offers access to various results reporting from lab and radiology, and even communicates with patients?

    a. Clinical messaging

    b. Clinical decision support

    c. Document management system

    d. Registration—admission, discharge, transfer

237. The HIM director is performing a staffing analysis to determine the number of employees needed to prep, scan, index, and carry out quality control on scanned medical records. Given a turnaround time of 24 hours and an average number of 48,000 images to be captured and considering the benchmarks listed here, what is the least number of employees the department needs, with each employee working an eight-hour shift?

Benchmarks for Document Scanning Processes	
Function	Expectations per Worked Hour
Prepping	340–500 images
Scanning	1,200–2,400 images
Quality Control	1,600–2,000 images
Indexing	600–800 images

  a. 25 employees

  b. 36 employees

  c. 36.1 employees

  d. 37 employees

238. A collection of data that is organized so its contents can be used to create reports and identify trends in the data is called a:

  a. Dashboard

  b. Database

  c. File

  d. Data table

239. Tom is the Coding Manager and has been in meetings with the HIM Director and Chief Financial Officer to determine different methods that would decrease the amount of time it takes to completely code a health record after the patient has been discharged. He is recommending a particular information system that performs part of its activities while the patient is still admitted and then is updated once the patient is discharged in order to improve efficiency to get claims submitted in a timely manner. This system is referred to as:

  a. ROI

  b. Transcription

  c. CAC

  d. CDI

240. What is the term for health records maintained by patients or their families?

  a. Electronic health records

  b. Mixed-media records

  c. Personal health records

  d. Longitudinal health records

241. What sets the acceptable level of quantity and quality for each function of a job?

  a. Performance standards

  b. Position descriptions

  c. Job procedures

  d. Job evaluation

242. The following table shows the LOS for a sample of 11 discharged patients. Using the data listed, calculate the range.

Patient	Length of Stay
1	1
2	3
3	5
4	3
5	2
6	29
7	3
8	4
9	2
10	1
11	2

a. 29

b. 1

c. 5

d. 28

243. Which application uses statistical techniques to determine the likelihood of certain events occurring together?

a. Predictive modeling

b. Standard deviation

c. T-test

d. Serial numbering

244. The following question was typed into the system: How many patients were discharged on November 12, 20XX? This is an example of what type of query?

a. Data manipulation language

b. Structured query language

c. Query by example

d. Natural language query

245. The generic formula for calculating rate of occurrence is used to calculate hospital-acquired infections in an intensive care unit in a given month. If the number of hospital-acquired infections is the numerator, the denominator would be the:

a. Number of patients who died of infection

b. Number of deaths in the ICU

c. Number of discharges (including deaths) of ICU patients

d. Total number of hospital discharges

246. A hospital allows the use of the copy functionality in its EHR system for documentation purposes. The hospital has established explicit policies that define when the copy function may be used. Which of the following would be the best approach for conducting a retrospective analysis to determine if hospital copy policies are being followed?

    a. Randomly audit EHR documentation for patients readmitted within 30 days.

    b. Survey practitioners to determine if they are following hospital policy.

    c. Institute an in-service program for all hospital personnel.

    d. Observe the documentation practices of all clinical personnel.

247. This type of data display tool is used to illustrate frequency distributions of continuous variables, such as age or length of stay (LOS).

    a. Bar graph

    b. Histogram

    c. Pie chart

    d. Scatter diagram

248. A database contains two tables: physicians and patients. If a physician may be linked to many patients and patients may only be related to one physician, what is the cardinality of the relationship between the two tables?

    a. One-to-one

    b. One-to-many

    c. Many-to-many

    d. One-to-two

249. Due to an influenza epidemic in Smithtown, the hospital is almost at full capacity. Which information system would be used to efficiently manage resources such as personnel, beds, and appointments of surgeries and CT scans, to coordinate equipment and staff as needed?

    a. Registration—admission, discharge, transfer

    b. Financial

    c. Scheduling

    d. Administrative

250. An EHR system is programmed by the vendor not to release certain patient data because it is considered proprietary to the vendor and a healthcare organization. The vendor is protecting its own business interests above that of the patient. This is an example of:

    a. Continuity of care record

    b. Graphic user interface

    c. HIPAA security breach

    d. Health information blocking

251. What trend can be summarized from the line plot shown in the chart?

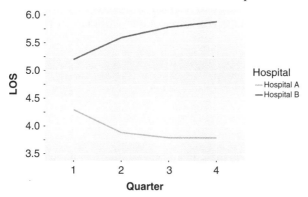

a. The length of stay has increased for hospital A and decreased for hospital B since the first quarter.

b. The length of stay for both hospitals decreased during the third quarter.

c. The length of stay has decreased for hospital A and increased for hospital B since the first quarter.

d. The length of stay for both hospitals increased during the third quarter.

252. A method that has been developed for presenting a variety of data on a single display in an easy-to-read format is called a:

a. Graph

b. Dashboard

c. Table

d. Data visualization

253. An HIM professional was conducting an audit to evaluate the timeframes for the administration of painkillers in surgical patients, and the medication administration record would be reviewed. The medication administration record would be found within which clinical software?

a. Nursing

b. Laboratory

c. Radiology

d. Pharmacy

254. What type of data mining technique would be used to group diagnoses?

a. Association rule learning

b. Anomaly detection

c. Regression analysis

d. Classification analysis

255. What term is used for a centralized database that captures, sorts, and processes patient data and then sends it back to the user?

a. Clinical data repository

b. Data exchange standard

c. Central processor

d. Digital system

256. Dr. Jones comes into the HIM department and requests that the HIM director provide a list of all of his patients from the previous year in which the principal diagnosis of myocardial infarction was indicated. Which index would the HIM director query from to provide Dr. Jones with this information?

    a. Disease index

    b. Master patient index

    c. Operative index

    d. Physician index

257. What elements would you change in the following graph to make the visualization more effective?

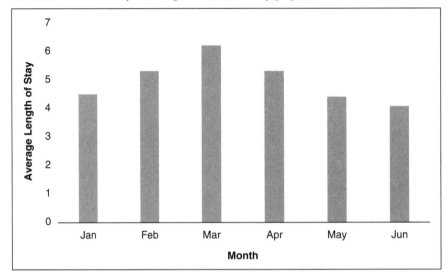

    a. Present the data in a vertical orientation

    b. Use a dot plot

    c. Remove the color

    d. Present the data as a line plot

258. The distribution in this curve is:

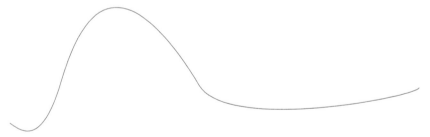

    a. Normal

    b. Bimodal

    c. Skewed left

    d. Skewed right

259. In January, Community Hospital had 57 discharges from its medicine unit. Four patients developed urinary tract infections while in the hospital. What is the hospital-acquired infection rate for the medicine unit for January?

    a. 0.07%

    b. 2.17%

    c. 7%

    d. 217%

260. The HIM director is on the design team for the CPOE system. During a user interface design session, a sample of the electronic system is demonstrated. Two of the physicians are concerned about the overuse of alerts. What problem could the alert feature pose in the new system?

    a. Unnecessary alerts can lead to clinicians ignoring other important alerts.

    b. Alerts make order entry difficult.

    c. Physicians do not like to be reminded how to treat patients.

    d. The Joint Commission discourages an alert system.

261. Prior to the implementation of the new EHR, the HIM manager is working with the IT analyst in order to improve departmental workflows. They are using structural metadata. This type of data can be used to create which of the following?

    a. Dataflow diagrams

    b. Data mapping

    c. Data audit

    d. Data architecture

262. Dr. Kotter treats highly unusual medical cases requiring many laboratory, radiology, and other diagnostic tests. Hospital administration wants to determine if additional facilities, personnel, and equipment are needed to meet current and future community demands. Which information system would be helpful in this scenario?

    a. Decision support system

    b. Registration—admission, discharge, transfer

    c. Clinical documentation improvement

    d. Executive information system

263. Which component of the EHR is designed to track and report outbreaks of infectious diseases and childhood immunization levels to public health officials?

    a. Population health

    b. Continuity of care record

    c. Results reporting

    d. Health information exchange

264. Kelly, the CDI specialist, is evaluating the information used by the coding professionals when they need to code various surgeries. She is particularly interested in the time lag between the actual surgical procedure and the determination of the pathology diagnosis. In which information system would the data element "principal procedure" be found?

    a. Transcription system

    b. Encoder/grouper

    c. Data quality indicator

    d. Tumor registry

265. In which type of health information exchange architectural model does the entity operate much like an application service provider (ASP) or bank vault?

    a. Consolidated

    b. Federated—consistent databases

    c. Federated—inconsistent databases

    d. Switch

266. Community Memorial Hospital discharged nine patients on April 1. The length of stay for each patient is shown in the following table. What is the median length of stay for this group of patients?

Patient	Length of Stay, in Days
A	1
B	5
C	3
D	3
E	8
F	8
G	8
H	9
I	9

    a. 5 days

    b. 6 days

    c. 8 days

    d. 9 days

267. Last year, 73,249 people died from diabetes mellitus in the United States. The total number of deaths from all causes was 2,443,387, and the total population was 288,356,713. Calculate the proportionate mortality ratio for diabetes mellitus.

    a. 0.003

    b. 10.94

    c. 0.09

    d. 3.0

268. In what condition is it more suitable to present data as a table instead of a graph?

   a. When the trend and the exact numeric value are important to the interpretation

   b. When the trend in values is most important

   c. When it is required to know the exact numeric value of a variable

   d. When the exact numeric value is not important to an interpretation

269. Which of the following basic services provided by a health information exchange (HIE) entity matches identifying information to an individual?

   a. Consent management

   b. Person identification

   c. Record locator

   d. Identity management

270. What type of system would look for contraindications between two medications, such as Warfarin (Coumadin) and ibuprofen, that could increase bleeding?

   a. Laboratory

   b. Radiology

   c. Pharmacy

   d. Nursing

271. Allowing different health information systems to work together within and across organizational boundaries is referred to as:

   a. Telehealth

   b. Interoperability

   c. Informatics

   d. Interfaces

272. Providing a process's policy and procedure guide to a user who has never used the information system and then asking the user to perform the process could be used in what type of testing?

   a. Application

   b. Documentation

   c. Volume

   d. Acceptance

273. The process of taking what is known at the highest level of understanding and working downward to identify the underlying causes for the high-level observation is called:

   a. Dashboard

   b. Slicing and dicing

   c. Data analytics

   d. Data visualization

274. What conclusions can you draw from the graph displayed below?

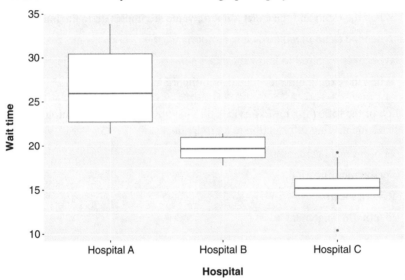

a. The hospitals have equal variance.

b. Hospital A has the greatest value and greatest variance.

c. Hospital B presents with outliers.

d. Hospital C has the smallest range of values.

275. Which of the following is an example of an activity that a patient may complete using a patient portal?

a. Bedside nursing care

b. Appointment scheduling

c. Direct patient care

d. Emergency care records

276. Which of the following basic services provided by an HIE entity identifies participating users and systems?

a. Identity management

b. Person identification

c. Registry and directory

d. Secure data transport

277. Algorithms are used to match duplicate patients in which the following information systems?

a. Decision support system

b. Executive information system

c. Master patient index system

d. Grouping system

278. In order to better prepare for hurricane season, Sunshine Hospital uses a variety of statistical models to help them figure out how to streamline the admissions process for emergency patients, determine what type of backup generators would meet their needs during a blackout, and determine which additional clinical staff will be needed during future disasters. This type of analytics is referred to as

    a. Simplistic

    b. Descriptive

    c. Diagnostic

    d. Prescriptive

279. An HIM professional takes data on denials that have been received by the healthcare facility over the past year. After manipulating the data, she learns that patients of Dr. Smith account for 30 percent of all denials. She schedules a meeting with Dr. Smith to discuss the matter. What process is the HIM professional conducting?

    a. Data informatics

    b. Data use

    c. Data analytics

    d. Data management

280. Data mining is a process that involves which of the following?

    a. Using reports to measure outcomes

    b. Using sophisticated computer technology to sort through an entity's data to identify unusual patterns

    c. Producing summary reports for management to run the daily activities of the healthcare entity

    d. Producing detailed reports to track productivity

281. If the medical office manager wanted to compare the amount of time it takes for a patient to be seen by a physician versus a nurse practitioner, which information system would be helpful in this analysis?

    a. Materials management system

    b. Practice management system

    c. Facilities management system

    d. Executive information system

282. What type of graph is the following, which is used to present the frequency distribution of a single numeric variable?

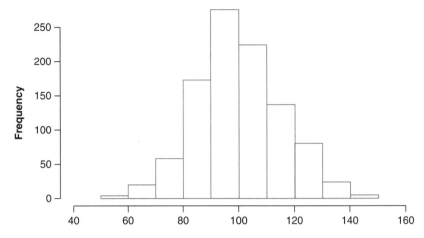

a. Box plot

b. Bar plot

c. Histogram

d. Line plot

283. Ethel is the QI Coordinator preparing for information governance implementation and additional quality reporting from the EHR system but has found gaps, inconsistent content, and incomplete data in the patient records. The HIM Manager recommends to her an information system that can be used to improve the communication between physicians and HIM staff to clarify information in the health record to improve its quality by making it more complete and accurate. This system is referred to as:

a. ROI

b. Transcription

c. CAC

d. CDI

284. The MPI has had numerous errors in which the last name field is filled with a date of birth. What is a preventive control that may help this situation?

a. An edit allowing only alphabetic entries could be added to the name field.

b. A report could be run showing which name fields had a number in them, and those errors could be fixed.

c. A report could be run showing which staff member entered the numeric data in the last name field; the supervisor could then discuss with the staff.

d. An audit could be performed to validate the issue.

285. In order to be properly evaluated, EHRs must be judged against measurable and objective criteria. In the healthcare and IT industries, these criteria are often referred to as

a. standards

b. benchmarks

c. norms

d. conditions

286. The term used to describe breaking data elements into the level of detail needed to retrieve the data is:

    a. Normalization

    b. Data definitions

    c. Primary key

    d. A database management system

287. What initiative has the ONC been driving through the escalation of technology and implementation and optimization of EHRs?

    a. Health information exchange

    b. False Claims Act

    c. HIPAA

    d. EMTALA

288. Consumer informatics is focused on:

    a. Consumer activation

    b. Information structures and processes

    c. Personalized medicine

    d. Engagement

289. If a health plan analyst wanted to determine if the readmission rates for two hospitals were statistically different, what is the null hypothesis?

    a. The readmission rates are not equal.

    b. The readmission rates are equal.

    c. The readmission rate for one hospital is larger than that of the other.

    d. The readmission rate for one hospital is smaller than that of the other.

290. Fifty percent of patients treated at our facilities have Medicare as their primary payer. This is an example of what type of information?

    a. Patient-specific

    b. Expert knowledge

    c. Comparative

    d. Aggregate

291. The probability of making a Type I error based on a particular set of data is called the:

    a. Sampling value

    b. Hypothesis test

    c. A-probability

    d. P-value

292. What must be in place to enhance the retrieval process for scanned documents?

    a. Electronic signature

    b. Indexing system

    c. RFID device

    d. Table of contents

293. As you continue the research on the COVID-19 pandemic impact on ABC Hospital, you've found that there is a higher mortality rate in COVID-19 patients due to cerebrovascular accidents. The autopsies show all of these patients suffered from many microinfarcts. What type of data analytics is being performed in this scenario?

    a. diagnostic analytics

    b. prescriptive analytics

    c. predictive analytics

    d. descriptive analytics

294. Laboratory data are successfully transmitted back and forth from Community Hospital to three local physician clinics. This successful transmission is dependent on which of the following standards?

    a. X12N

    b. LOINC

    c. RxNorm

    d. DICOM

295. When describing the typical length of stay for patients admitted for congestive heart failure, which is the most appropriate measure of central tendency when there are a number of long stay outliers?

    a. Minimum

    b. Mean

    c. Median

    d. Mode

Revenue Cycle Management

296. David was admitted to the hospital following an automobile accident in which he suffered a fractured femur. Two days after surgery to repair the fracture, he developed pneumonia and was transferred to the ICU. Because the pneumonia was not present at the time of admission to the hospital, it is considered a:

a. Healthcare-associated infection

b. Hospital sickness

c. Community-acquired infection

d. Community sickness

297. The goal of revenue integrity is to produce a claim that is _____.

a. Clean, complete, and compliant

b. Complete, accurate, and timely

c. Clean, timely, and includes modifiers

d. Compliant, clean, and includes diagnosis

298. What is the maximum number of days that Medicare will cover skilled nursing facility inpatient care?

a. 21

b. 30

c. 60

d. 100

299. Which term is used for retrospective reimbursement charges submitted by a provider for each service rendered?

a. Fee-for-service

b. Deductible

c. Actuarial

d. Prospective

300. George Benson, age 72, was admitted to the hospital on March 1st and was discharged on May 15th. He has not met his benefit period deductible. He also has not used his reserve days. If the current Medicare rates for the patient's responsibility are:

   ○ Benefit period deductible: $1,364

   ○ Days 61-90: $341 per day

   ○ Days 91-150: $682 per day

What is George's financial responsibility for this inpatient visit?

a. $1,364

b. $6,479

c. $6,820

d. $25,916

301. A patient is treated in observation and fell out of his bed. An x-ray shows a femoral fracture. The patient is admitted as an inpatient to treat the hip fracture. What is the POA indicator for the fracture for the inpatient admission?

    a. Y

    b. N

    c. U

    d. W

302. The insurance verification process involves confirming the patient is a member of the insurance plan and this fact is communicated to the provider. Which of the following statements involving insurance verification reflects the most common time when insurance verification occurs for an unscheduled patient?

    a. Prior to medical screening

    b. During or directly after preregistration

    c. After the patient is released from care

    d. After medical screening

303. Which of the following assists with identifying issues involving data elements to ensure clean claims to be submitted to the payers?

    a. Clinical documentation improvement program

    b. Claims management follow up software

    c. APC grouper or claim scrubber software

    d. Order tracking and management system

304. When radiological and other procedures that include professional and technical components are paid as a lump sum that is to be divided between the physician and the healthcare facility, this is called a:

    a. Global payment

    b. Professional payment

    c. Unbundled payment

    d. Fee-for-service payment

305. If an organization has an average daily gross patient service revenue of $230,000 along with 120 patient preregistered encounters, 150 scheduled encounters, and $100,000 in gross dollars in discharged, not final billed accounts, what is the DNFB rate?

    a. 43.5%

    b. 52.1%

    c. 2.3%

    d. 80.0%

306. Determinations of medical necessity reflect the efficient and cost-effective application of patient care for which of the following?

    a. Positive patient interactions

    b. Previous medical conditions

    c. Physician restrictions

    d. Diagnostic testing

307. Being excluded from participating in Medicare or other federal programs is significant because _____.

    a. The government is the largest purchaser of healthcare services in the country

    b. Jailtime always accompanies exclusion

    c. Those excluded are covicted of fraud, not abuse

    d. Facilties or individuals excluded from federal programs must undergo extensive offender training

308. When a payer questions a clinical aspect of an admission, such as length of stay of the admission, the level of service, if the encounter meets medical necessity parameters, the site of the service, or if clinical validation is not passed, this is called a/an:

    a. Administrative denial

    b. Clinical trial

    c. Clinical denial

    d. Administrative trial

309. Which of the following occurs when the organization assumes potential losses associated with a given risk and makes plans to cover the financial consequences.

    a. Corporate integrity agreements (CIAs)

    b. Risk assessment

    c. Risk retention

    d. Contingency planning

310. A newborn is treated for pulmonary valve stenosis, with stretching of the valve opening accomplished via a percutaneous balloon pulmonary valvuloplasty. In ICD-10-PCS, what root operation would be coded for this procedure?

    a. Alteration

    b. Dilation

    c. Repair

    d. Restriction

311. If the whistleblower is an employee, which of the following actions can the employer take against the employee?

    a. Termination

    b. Suspension

    c. No action is taken

    d. Demotion

312. The following are the most common reasons for claim denials *except*:

    a. Billing noncovered services

    b. Lack of support for medical necessity

    c. Untimely filing

    d. Coverage not in effect for date of service

313. _____ results when someone without authorization obtains healthcare services under someone else's name or purchases insurance coverage based on someone else's clean bill of health.

    a. Red Flags Rule

    b. Medical identity theft

    c. HIPAA Violation

    d. Whistleblowing

314. If your hospital's net days in accounts receivable is 62 and the local peer hospital's net days in accounts receivable is 46, your hospital's A/R value compared to the local peer hospital would be considered _____.

    a. Favorable

    b. Unfavorable

    c. Average

    d. Insignificant

315. Which of the following individuals assists in communicating with and educating medical staff as part of the CDI program?

    a. Medical officer

    b. Chief of staff

    c. Department chairperson

    d. Physician champion

316. Which of the following tools is typically used to support the processes in the back end of the revenue cycle?

    a. Chargemaster maintenance software

    b. Preregistration

    c. Charge capture

    d. Automated claim status and cash posting

317. Improving account collections while creating a positive consumer experience can be accomplished through a recognized method of _____.

    a. Denying service at the pre-registration process

    b. Electronic payment options through a patient portal

    c. Auditing the EOB with the patient to determine if payment is necessary

    d. Using a threshold to determine account review and then sending account to third-party collection agency

318. A patient is admitted for an appendectomy. Postoperatively, the patient develops a pulmonary embolism. What is the POA indicator for the pulmonary embolism?

    a. Y

    b. N

    c. U

    d. W

319. Which of the following reimbursement methods pays providers according to charges that are calculated before the healthcare services are rendered?

    a. Fee-for-service reimbursement

    b. Prospective payment

    c. Retrospective payment

    d. Resource-based payment

320. A patient has HIV with disseminated candidiasis. What is the correct code assignment?

B20	Human immunodeficiency virus [HIV] disease
B37.0	Candidal stomatitis
	Oral thrush
B37.7	Candidal sepsis
	Disseminated candidiasis
	Systemic candidiasis
B37.89	Other sites of candidiasis
	Candidal osteomyelitis

    a. B20, B37.0

    b. B37.7, B20

    c. B20, B37.7

    d. B20, B37.89, B37.7

321. A patient was admitted for removal of the left lobe of the liver via laparotomy due to metastasis from a colon carcinoma. What is the correct ICD-10-PCS procedure code for this operation?

Section	Body System	Root Operation	Body Part	Approach	Device	Qualifier
Medical and Surgical	Hepatobiliary System and Pancreas	Excision	Liver, Left Lobe	Open	No Device	No Qualifier
0	F	B	2	0	Z	Z

Section	Body System	Root Operation	Body Part	Approach	Device	Qualifier
Medical and Surgical	Hepatobiliary System and Pancreas	Excision	Liver, Left Lobe	Percutaneous Endoscopic	No Device	No Qualifier
0	F	B	2	4	Z	Z

Section	Body System	Root Operation	Body Part	Approach	Device	Qualifier
Medical and Surgical	Hepatobiliary System and Pancreas	Resection	Liver, Left Lobe	Open	No Device	No Qualifier
0	F	T	2	0	Z	Z

Section	Body System	Root Operation	Body Part	Approach	Device	Qualifier
Medical and Surgical	Hepatobiliary System and Pancreas	Resection	Liver, Left Lobe	Percutaneous Endoscopic	No Device	No Qualifier
0	F	T	2	4	Z	Z

a. 0FB20ZZ

b. 0FB24ZZ

c. 0FT20ZZ

d. 0FT24ZZ

322. A 65-year-old woman was admitted to the hospital. She was diagnosed with sepsis secondary to methicillin susceptible *Staphylococcus aureus* and abdominal pain secondary to diverticulitis of the colon. What is the correct code assignment?

A41.01	Sepsis due to Methicillin susceptible *Staphylococcus aureus*
A41.89	Other specified sepsis
A41.9	Sepsis, unspecified organism
B95.61	Methicillin susceptible *Staphylococcus aureus* infection as the cause of diseases classified elsewhere
K57.32	Diverticulitis of large intestine without perforation or abscess without bleeding
R10.9	Unspecified abdominal pain

a. A41.89, K57.32, R10.9

b. A41.01, K57.32

c. A41.89, K57.32, B95.61

d. A41.9, K57.32

323. A patient was admitted to the hospital and diagnosed with Type 1 diabetic gangrene. What is the correct code assignment?

E08.52	Diabetes mellitus due to underlying condition with diabetic peripheral angiopathy with gangrene
E10.52	Type 1 diabetes mellitus with diabetic peripheral angiopathy with gangrene
E10.8	Type 1 diabetes mellitus with unspecified complications
I96	Gangrene, not elsewhere classified

   a. E08.52, I96

   b. E10.52, I96

   c. E10.8

   d. E10.52

324. Which of the following is considered a type of registration issue affecting the revenue cycle?

   a. Patient registered with more than one medical record number

   b. Accurately recording the patient's guarantor and employer information

   c. Excessive wait time for patients in the registration area

   d. Completion of insurance verification

325. In which of the following documents can regulatory requirements and revisions regarding national and local coverage determinations (NCDs and LCDs) be found?

   a. Medicare billing manuals

   b. Official ICD-10 coding guidelines

   c. Local managed care contract language

   d. Notice of privacy practices

326. A patient with a diagnosis of ventral hernia is admitted to undergo a laparotomy with ventral hernia repair. The patient undergoes a laparotomy and develops bradycardia. The operative site is closed without the repair of the hernia. What is the correct code assignment?

I97.191	Other postprocedural cardiac functional disturbances following other surgery
K43.9	Ventral hernia without obstruction or gangrene
R00.1	Bradycardia, unspecified
Z53.09	Procedure and treatment not carried out because of other contraindication

Section	Body System	Root Operation	Body Part	Approach	Device	Qualifier
Medical and Surgical	Anatomical Regions, General	Inspection	Peritoneal Cavity	Open	No Device	No Qualifier
0	W	J	G	0	Z	Z

Section	Body System	Root Operation	Body Part	Approach	Device	Qualifier
Medical and Surgical	Anatomical Regions, General	Repair	Abdominal Wall	Open	No Device	No Qualifier
0	W	Q	F	0	Z	Z

a. K43.9, R00.1, Z53.09, 0WJG0ZZ

b. K43.9, I97.191, R00.1, 0WJG0ZZ

c. K43.9, 0WQF0ZZ

d. K43.9, Z53.09, 0WQF0ZZ

327. Assign the correct CPT code for the following: A 63-year-old female had a temporal artery biopsy completed in the outpatient surgical center.

a. 32408, Core needle biopsy, lung or mediastinum, percutaneous, including imaging guidance, when performed

b. 37609, Ligation or biopsy, temporal artery

c. 20206, Biopsy, muscle, percutaneous needle

d. 31629, Bronchoscopy, rigid or flexible, including fluoroscopic guidance, when performed; with transbronchial needle aspiration biopsy(s), trachea, main stem and/or lobar bronchus(i)

328. Which of the following processes are financial counselors typically responsible for?

a. Determining whether the patient is eligible for charity care

b. Verifying whether the patient's insurance plan is in network or out of network

c. Determining whether scheduled services will be covered by the insurance plan

d. Understanding which procedures require preauthorization

329. The insurance verification process involves confirming the patient is a member of the insurance plan communicated to the provider. Which of the following describes the most common time when insurance verification occurs for an unscheduled patient?

    a. Prior to medical screening

    b. During or directly after preregistration

    c. After the patient is released from care

    d. After medical screening

330. A patient was admitted to the hospital with symptoms of a stroke and secondary diagnoses of chronic obstructive pulmonary disease (COPD) and hypertension. The patient was subsequently discharged from the hospital with a principal diagnosis of cerebral vascular accident and secondary diagnoses of catheter-associated urinary tract infection, COPD, and hypertension. Which of the following diagnoses should *not* be reported as POA?

    a. Catheter-associated urinary tract infection

    b. Cerebral vascular accident

    c. COPD

    d. Hypertension

331. Assign the correct CPT code for the following: A 58-year-old male was seen in the outpatient surgical center for insertion of a self-contained inflatable penile prosthesis for impotence.

    a. 54401, Insertion of penile prosthesis; inflatable (self-contained)

    b. 54405, Insertion of multicomponent, inflatable penile prosthesis, including placement of pump, cylinders, and reservoir

    c. 54440, Plastic operation of penis for injury

    d. 54400, Insertion of penile prosthesis, non-inflatable (semi-rigid)

332. Assign the correct CPT code for the following procedure: Patient is admitted to move the skin pocket for their pacemaker.

    a. 33223, Relocation of skin pocket for implantable defibrillator

    b. 33210, Insertion or replacement of temporary transvenous single chamber cardiac electrode or pacemaker catheter (separate procedure)

    c. 33212, Insertion of pacemaker pulse generator only; with existing single lead

    d. 33222, Relocation of skin pocket for pacemaker

333. Patient accounting is reporting an increase in national coverage decisions (NCDs), and local coverage determinations (LCDs) failed edits in observation accounts. Which of the following departments will be tasked to resolve this issue?

    a. Utilization management

    b. Patient access

    c. Health information management

    d. Patient accounts

334. Which of the following is typically the responsibility of the contract management team?

    a. Marketing of new services to affiliated clinics

    b. Determining whether services are set up to reflect the proper CPT/HCPCS codes and revenue codes on the billing claim

    c. Analyzing whether discount rates are providing financial incentives that steer the patient population

    d. Conducting a SWOT analysis to maintain the facility's competitive advantage

335. Patient accounts has submitted a report to the revenue cycle team detailing $100,000 of outpatient accounts that are failing NCD edits. All attempts to clear the edits have failed. There are no ABNs on file for these accounts. Based only on this information, the revenue cycle team should:

    a. Bill the patients for these accounts

    b. Contact the patients to obtain an ABN

    c. Write off the accounts to contractual allowances

    d. Write off the failed charges to bad debt and bill Medicare for the clean charges

336. Under RBRVS, which elements are used to calculate a Medicare payment?

    a. Work value and extent of the physical exam

    b. Malpractice expenses and detail of the patient history

    c. Work value and practice expenses

    d. Practice expenses and review of systems

337. In reviewing a patient chart, the coder finds that the patient's chest x-ray is suggestive of chronic obstructive pulmonary disease (COPD). The attending physician mentions the x-ray finding in one progress note, but no medication, treatment, or further evaluation is provided. Which of the following actions should the coder take in this case?

    a. Query the attending physician and ask him to validate a diagnosis based on the chest x-ray results

    b. Code COPD because the documentation substantiates it

    c. Query the radiologist to determine whether the patient has COPD

    d. Assign a code from the abnormal findings to reflect the condition

338. Which of the following is most applicable to describing utilization management functions?

    a. Begins only after patient admission

    b. Provides criteria to monitor for the continued appropriateness of the supplies and patient convenience items

    c. Screens for the appropriate use of hospital services and resources

    d. Applies criteria to determine medications that should be prescribed

339. Using the information provided, if the physician is a non-PAR who accepts assignment, how much can he or she expect to be reimbursed by Medicare?

> Physician's normal charge = $340
> Medicare Fee Schedule = $300
> Patient has met his deductible

   a. $228

   b. $240

   c. $285

   d. $300

340. When a procedure is performed by visualizing the operative field via an orifice, without using instrumentation, which ICD-10-PCS approach value is correct?

   a. Open

   b. Percutaneous endoscopic

   c. External

   d. Via natural or artificial opening endoscopic

341. Hospital-issued notices of noncoverage (HINNs) can be issued at any of the following times *except*:

   a. Prior to admission

   b. At admission

   c. At any point during the hospital stay

   d. After discharge

342. Understanding adjustments in payment to the provider and then utilizing the information to determine subsequent revenue audit and recovery efforts initiate from which of the following?

   a. Remittance advice

   b. Claim form 837

   c. Adverse determination

   d. Accounts receivable

Use the following figure for questions 343 and 344:

ABC Premiere Health Plan	
MEMBER	**POLICY NUMBER**
JANE B.	WHITE HS 123456 7890
GROUP	
STATE	
TYPE	EFFEC 01012005
EFFEC 01012005	
EMPLOYEE-ONLY	
SEND ALL BILLS TO:	
ABC Premiere Health Plan	
1500 Primrose Path	
Flowerville, XX 12345	

343. From the figure, determine whether the plan covers Gill F. White, Jane's spouse.

    a. No, the card states "Employee-Only"

    b. Yes, the policy number includes "S"

    c. Yes, the group is "State"

    d. Cannot be determined

344. From the figure, determine which entity that has purchased the insurance policy.

    a. 1234567890

    b. STATE

    c. ABC Premiere Health Plan

    d. Jane B. White

345. When attempting to build patient relations and customer service in the revenue cycle related to the patient's financial obligations, providers should focus which of the following approaches?

    a. Consumer-centric approach

    b. Patient engagement approach

    c. Transparency approach

    d. Payment variance approach

346. A clinical documentation improvement (CDI) program facilitates accurate coding and helps coders avoid:

    a. NCCI edits

    b. Upcoding

    c. Coding without a completed face sheet

    d. Assumption coding

347. Which of the following is a reason to deliver a hospital-issued notice of noncoverage (HINN) to a Medicare beneficiary?

    a. Service is not medically necessary

    b. Service was preauthorized

    c. Service was delivered in the most appropriate setting

    d. Service is provided in the emergency room

348. Reviewing claims to ensure appropriate coding for deserved payments is one method of:

    a. Achieving legitimate optimization

    b. Improving documentation

    c. Ensuring compliance

    d. Using data monitors

349. Which of the following is an example of internal medical identity theft?

    a. Sue in her role as a patient registration clerk uses a patient's insurance information to see a specialist for cosmetic surgery.

    b. Joe uses a patient's information obtained through hacking the healthcare facility system.

    c. Joan, an ICU nurse accesses the record of the patient she is currently treating.

    d. Bob introduces a virus into the facility's health information system.

350. The federal government is determined to lower the overall payments to physicians. To incur the least administrative work, which of the following elements of the physician payment system would the government reduce?

    a. Conversion factor

    b. RVU

    c. GPCI

    d. Weighted discount

351. The provider staff who are involved with communicating adverse determinations to patients and their families are considered:

    a. Financial counselors

    b. Utilization management staff

    c. Registration staff

    d. Patient financial services staff

352. Part of the coding supervisor's responsibility is to review accounts that have not been final billed due to errors. One of the accounts on the list is a same-day procedure. Upon review, the coding supervisor notices that the charge code on the bill was hard-coded. The ambulatory procedure coder added the same CPT code to the abstract. How should this error be corrected?

    a. Delete the code from the CDM because it should not be there.

    b. Refer the case to the chargemaster coordinator.

    c. Force a final bill on the accounts since the duplication will not affect the UB-04.

    d. Remove the code from the abstract and counsel the coder regarding CDM hard codes in this service.

353. Which of the following is true about the advance beneficiary notification of noncoverage?

    a. Estimates patient's financial out-of-pocket financial responsibility

    b. Supports patients with financial assistance applications

    c. May be issued when an inpatient service has been regarded noncovered due to medical necessity

    d. Required to be issued when outpatient service is considered not likely to be covered by Medicare

354. In the HHPPS system, which home healthcare services are consolidated into a single payment to home health agencies?

    a. Home health aide visits, routine and nonroutine medical supplies, durable medical equipment

    b. Routine and nonroutine medical supplies, durable medical equipment, medical social services

    c. Nursing and therapy services, routine and nonroutine medical supplies, home health aide visits

    d. Nursing and therapy services, durable medical equipment, medical social services

355. The coder assigned separate codes for individual tests when a combination code exists. This is an example of which of the following?

    a. Upcoding

    b. Complex coding

    c. Query

    d. Unbundling

356. Community Hospital implemented a clinical document improvement (CDI) program six months ago. The goal of the program was to improve clinical documentation to support quality of care, data quality, and HIM coding accuracy. Which of the following would be best to ensure that everyone understands the importance of this program?

    a. Request that the CEO write a memorandum to all hospital staff

    b. Give the chairperson of the CDI committee authority to fire employees who do not improve their clinical documentation

    c. Include ancillary clinical staff and medical staff in the process

    d. Request a letter of support from the Joint Commission

357. A financial counselor assumes responsibility for which of the following?

    a. Ensuring appropriate and timely care is provided

    b. Identifies barriers to patient progression through healthcare services

    c. Connects with patients after they leave the provider

    d. Determines sources of payment for healthcare services rendered

358. The accounts receivable collection cycle involves the time from:

    a. Discharge to receipt of the money

    b. Admission to billing the account

    c. Admission to deposit in the bank

    d. Billing of the account to deposit in the bank

359. The physician marked his superbill for a moderate level of care for every patient based on the concept that historically, on average, his reimbursements for all patients have been at that level. Additionally, he considered that he would save time, both for himself and his biller, by not having to figure out the actual time spent and level of complexity of medical decision-making required to assign the actual CPT E/M level for the case. His biller is curious and asks you whether this is appropriate. Your response is:

    a. Systematic, intentional miscoding of cases is fraud, and he should not do this.

    b. This is a great time saver, and you will consider doing the same for ED cases in the hospital.

    c. Although this is a violation of CPT coding rules, it will not affect his reimbursement, so it is okay.

    d. This is abuse of the reimbursement system, and he should not do this.

360. The lead coder in the HIM department is an acknowledged coding expert and is the go-to person in the healthcare entity for coding guidance. As the HIM director you learn that she is not following proper coding guidelines and her coding practices are not compliant. As the HIM director, the best steps to take would be which of the following?

    a. Report to the coder to the OIG and terminate the coder

    b. Notify the compliance officer and suspend the employee

    c. Review the coding errors and counsel the employee

    d. Ignore the coding errors

361. To meet the definition of an inpatient rehabilitation facility (IRF), facilities must have an inpatient population with at least a specified percentage of patients with certain conditions. Which of the following conditions is counted in the definition?

    a. Brain injury

    b. Chronic myelogenous leukemia

    c. Acute myocardial infarction

    d. Cancer

362. You are the director of patient access services. Mary Smith, 35, is calling you because she received a bill from the hospital for services rendered last month that her insurance did not reimburse. She also has an EOB from her insurance company. Mary does not use your hospital, has never been there, and tells you that her primary care physician is associated with an entirely different hospital. Upon review of the patient file, you confirm that Mary's patient data is correct in your system. What is the problem, and what should you do?

    a. Mary is confused and does not remember the visit. You should ask to speak to a family member who can explain the situation to her.

    b. Mary is trying to get out of paying the bill. You should refer her to patient financial services and transfer the call.

    c. Mary is possibly a victim of medical identity theft. You should alert your security and compliance departments.

    d. Mary is confused. You should offer to send her the medical records to demonstrate that she was there.

363. The process in which a healthcare entity addresses the provider documentation issues of legibility, completeness, clarity, consistency, and precision is called:

    a. Query process

    b. Release of information process

    c. Coding process

    d. Case-finding process

364. Which of the following terms describes the requirement for a healthcare provider to obtain permission from the health insurer in order to provide predefined services to the patient?

    a. Preauthorization

    b. Coordination of benefits

    c. Informed consent

    d. Preassessment

365. Which of the following items are packaged under the Medicare hospital outpatient prospective payment system (OPPS)?

    a. Recovery room and medical visits

    b. Medical visits and supplies (other than pass-through)

    c. Anesthesia and ambulance services

    d. Supplies (other than pass-through) and recovery room

366. Gladys Johnson was admitted to the skilled nursing facility for 30 days. If the current Medicare coverage for SNF care is:

    First 20 days = 100% of approved amount

    Days 21-100 = all but $170.50 per day

    Beyond 100 days = Nothing

    What is Gladys' total financial responsibility for the SNF stay?

    a. $1,705.00

    b. $5,115.00

    c. $170.50

    d. Nothing, Medicare pays for all 30 days

367. The Red Flags Rule _____ an organization to implement a protection program that identifies warnings that alert the organization that potential identity theft has occurred or is occurring.

    a. Requires

    b. Does not require

    c. Sometimes requires

    d. Recommends as best practice

368. Who assumes the risk of loss in caring for a patient who is covered under a capitation contract?

    a. Patient

    b. Policy holder

    c. Payer

    d. Provider

369. Anywhere Hospital is implementing a new clinical documentation improvement (CDI) program. As part of the program, the clinical staff is educated on the components and procedures of the program. Which of the following would *not* be true about the CDI program?

    a. The need for postdischarge queries will be eliminated.

    b. Physicians will be consulted about nonspecific documentation while patients are still in-house.

    c. Effective communication between clinical staff and CDI specialist is vital.

    d. CDI reviewers will be on the inpatient units to review clinical documentation concurrently.

370. In a typical acute-care setting, the explanation of benefits, Medicare summary notice, and remittance advice documents (provided by the payer) are monitored in which revenue cycle area?

    a. Preclaims submission

    b. Claims processing

    c. Accounts receivable

    d. Claims reconciliation

371. There are several physicians on staff who continue to write "urosepsis" in the patient charts. The term "urosepsis" has no meaning in the ICD-10-CM code set. Coders repeatedly have to query the physicians to ask for a definitive diagnosis. What is the most efficient way to solve the problem?

    a. The HIM director should speak to the physicians and tell them to write "urinary tract infection" instead of "urosepsis."

    b. Patient financial services should meet with the physicians to educate them.

    c. CDI staff should be alert to this documentation issue so they can query the term while the patient is still in house, and the physicians should be counseled by the chief medical officer or CDI liaison regarding the correct documentation.

    d. The physicians should be placed on suspension until they learn to document correctly.

372. The health record review process and what other aspect allow for the highest level of quality in clinical documentation?

    a. Training on the revenue cycle

    b. Medical necessity

    c. Training on basics of coding

    d. Physician queries

373. The purpose of this program is to reduce improper Medicare payments and prevent future improper payments made on claims of healthcare services:

    a. Medicare provider analysis and review

    b. Recovery audit contractors

    c. Medicare Conditions of Participation

    d. Health Insurance Portability and Accountability Act

374. A payer has advised your hospital that it is auditing records from last year due to a suspected payment error. Your hospital's first action should be to:

    a. Review the contract to determine whether this is a violation of the look-back period clause

    b. Request a list of the records to be reviewed and make sure the payer is requesting records that are specifically associated with that payer only

    c. Ask the payer to specifically identify the suspected payment error

    d. Notify HIM of the request for release of information

375. Charges for items that must be reported separately but are used together, such as interventional radiology imaging and injection procedures are called:

    a. Insurance code mappings

    b. Charge codes

    c. Exploding charges

    d. Revenue Codes

376. Identity theft is primarily a financial crime. However, _____ can impact an individual's ability to obtain health care and health insurance coverage.

    a. The False Claims Act

    b. The Red Flags Rule

    c. Medical identity theft

    d. Whistleblowing

377. There has been a recent increase in errors regarding the posting of the admitting diagnosis. Correction of this error falls to the coding staff. With which department will HIM have to partner in order to identify and eliminate this recurring error?

    a. Patient access

    b. Patient financial services

    c. Case management

    d. Medical staff

378. With what agency may patients file a complaint if they suspect medical identity theft violations?

    a. Internal Revenue Service

    b. Office of Civil Rights

    c. Centers for Medicare and Medicaid Services

    d. Federal Trade Commission

379. A patient is scheduled for elective services, and preregistration has determined that insurance does not cover all of the reimbursement for the procedure. What does the registrar do first?

    a. Demand payment in advance

    b. Offer financial counseling services

    c. Cancel the services

    d. Call the physician to explain the situation

380. When someone without authorization obtains healthcare services under someone else's name or purchases insurance coverage based on someone else's clean bill of health, this is called:

    a. Red Flags Rule

    b. Medical identity theft

    c. HIPAA Violation

    d. Whistleblowing

381. A patient is admitted with coughing and fever. X-rays show bilateral pneumonia. She is not responding to antibiotics and is admitted to the ICU with severe sepsis. The physician documents that he is not sure whether the sepsis was present on admission or not. What is the POA indicator for the sepsis?

    a. Y

    b. N

    c. U

    d. W

382. An internal coding audit at Community Hospital shows that the cause of improper coding is lack of proper physician documentation to support reimbursement at the appropriate level. Coders have found that coding issues result because physician documentation needs clarification. The HIM department staff has met periodically with each clinical specialty to improve communication and provide targeted education, but documentation problems still persist. Which of the following actions would be the most reliable and consistent method to improve communication and documentation?

    a. Revise medical staff bylaws to include documentation requirements.

    b. Suspend medical staff privileges after a specified number of documentation problems have occurred.

    c. Implement a standardized physician query form so that coders can request clarification from physicians about documentation issues.

    d. Allow coders to make clinical judgments in the absence of physician documentation.

383. The facility's Medicare case-mix index has dropped, although other statistical measures appear constant. The CFO suspects coding errors. What type of coding quality review should be performed?

    a. Random audit

    b. Focused audit

    c. Compliance audit

    d. External audit

384. During a recent coding audit, the coding manager identified the following error made by a coder. The coder assigned the following codes for a female patient who was admitted for stress incontinence and a urethral suspension without mesh was performed:

| N39.3 | Stress incontinence (female) (male) |
| OTUD0JZ | Urethral suspension |

What error was made by the coder?

N23	Unspecified renal colic
N39.3	Stress incontinence (female) (male)
R32	Unspecified urinary incontinence

Section	Body System	Root Operation	Body Part	Approach	Device	Qualifier
Medical and Surgical	Urinary System	Reposition	Urethra	Open	No Device	No Qualifier
0	T	S	D	0	Z	Z

Section	Body System	Root Operation	Body Part	Approach	Device	Qualifier
Medical and Surgical	Urinary System	Supplement	Urethra	Open	Synthetic Substitute	No Qualifier
0	T	U	D	0	J	Z

    a. The coder assigned the correct diagnosis and procedure codes.

    b. The coder assigned the correct diagnosis code but assigned the incorrect root operation for the procedure.

    c. The coder assigned the correct procedure code but the incorrect diagnosis code.

    d. The coder assigned the correct diagnosis code but selected the incorrect device character for the procedure code.

385. All of the following are examples of identity theft red flags categories *except*:

    a. Alerts or notification from a consumer reporting agency

    b. Suspicious documents

    c. Alerts or notification from AHIMA

    d. Suspicious personally identifying information

386. The most recent coding audit has revealed a tendency to miss secondary diagnoses that would have increased the reimbursement for the case. Which of the following strategies would be most likely to correct this problem in the long term?

    a. Focused reviews on changes in MS-DRGs

    b. Facility top 10 to 15 DRGs by volume and charges

    c. Contracting with a larger consulting firm to do audits and education

    d. Development and implementation of a CDI program

387. Which of the following is the principal goal of internal auditing programs for billing and coding?

    a. Increase revenues

    b. Protect providers from sanctions or fines

    c. Improve patient care

    d. Limit unnecessary changes to the chargemaster

388. You are the coding manager and are completing a review of a new coder's work. The case facts are that the patient was treated in the emergency department for two forearm lacerations that were both repaired with simple closure. The new coder assigned one CPT code for the largest laceration. Which of the following would be the correct CPT code assignment for this case?

    a. One CPT code for the largest laceration

    b. Two CPT codes, one for each laceration

    c. One CPT code adding the lengths of the lacerations together

    d. One CPT code for the most complex closure

389. Which of the following requires financial institutions to develop written medical identity theft programs?

    a. HIPAA Security Rule

    b. HITECH Act

    c. Fair and Accurate Credit Transactions Act

    d. HIPAA Privacy and Security Rule

390. A patient is admitted to the hospital with shortness of breath and congestive heart failure. The patient undergoes intubation with mechanical ventilation. The final diagnoses documented by the attending physician are: Congestive heart failure, mechanical ventilation, and intubation. Which of the following actions should the coder take in this case?

    a. Code congestive heart failure, respiratory failure, mechanical ventilation, and intubation

    b. Query the attending physician as to the reason for the intubation and mechanical ventilation to add as a secondary diagnosis

    c. Query the attending physician about the adding the symptom of shortness of breath as a secondary diagnosis

    d. Code shortness of breath, congestive heart failure, mechanical ventilation, and intubation

391. Automated review efforts of recovery audit contractors (RAC) allow them to deny payments without ever reviewing a health record based on the information they gather without having access to the record. Which of the following would be an example of a potential denial based on information the RAC contractor would have without the health record?

    a. A coder assigning the wrong DRG for a patient

    b. Billing for two colonoscopies on the same day for the same Medicare beneficiary

    c. An inaccurate principal diagnosis

    d. A principal procedure code

392. Daniel's supervisor is requiring him to code inpatient Medicare charts with a diagnosis of pneumonia as having mechanical ventilation provided, whether or not the chart supports this. Daniel has voiced his concerns about this practice but nothing has changed. Daniel makes a call to the OIG to report this practice, and an audit is forthcoming. In this case, Daniel is acting as a(n) _____:

    a. Arbitrator

    b. Mediator

    c. Ombudsman

    d. Whistleblower

393. Which of the following payment methods reimburses healthcare providers in the form of lump sums for all healthcare services delivered to a patient for a specific illness?

    a. Managed fee-for-service

    b. Capitation

    c. Episode-of-care

    d. Point of service

394. Given of the following data elements in the charge master, which value will not transfer to the billing claim form?

Charge code	Charge code description	HCPCS code	Modifier	Revenue code	Price
760211	Direct admit to Observation	G0379		762	$1,179.00

    a. G0379

    b. 760211

    c. $1,179.00

    d. 762

395. The HHS OIG publishes a yearly work plan that outlines _____.

    a. A schedule of audits to be undertaken

    b. Proposed targets of reviews by geographic region

    c. Projects that are planned and the areas identified for review

    d. New compliance measures for public facilities

396. According to CPT, an endoscopy that is undertaken to the level of the midtransverse colon would be coded as a:

    a. Proctosigmoidoscopy

    b. Colonoscopy

    c. Sigmoidoscopy

    d. Anoscopy

397. Under the APC system, multiple procedures performed during the same surgical encounter are reimbursed at which of the following rates?

    a. All significant procedures receive full (100 percent) payment.

    b. The procedure in the highest APC receives full payment and the remaining procedures receive half (50 percent) payment.

    c. The procedure in the lowest APC receives full payment and the remaining procedures receive half (50 percent) payment.

    d. The procedure in the highest APC receives full payment and the remaining procedures receive seventy-five (75 percent) payment.

398. A Staghorn calculus of the left renal pelvis was treated earlier in the week by lithotripsy and is now removed via a percutaneous nephrostomy tube. What is the root operation performed for this procedure?

    a. Destruction

    b. Fragmentation

    c. Extraction

    d. Extirpation

399. Key clinical documents required for coding are defined by _____.

    a. The OIG

    b. The organizational coding compliance plan and departmental policies

    c. CMS

    d. The organization's CDI steering committee

400. Every CDI program should use which of the following important feedback tools for improvement and communication purposes.

    a. Metrics

    b. Committees

    c. Database

    d. Physician advisors

401. In Medicare's resource-based relative value scale payment system, which factor adjusts payments to physicians and health professionals for price differences among various parts of the country?

    a. Practice RVU

    b. Malpractice RVU

    c. Geographic practice cost index

    d. Conversion factor

402. The patient is admitted with acute MI and undergoes a coronary artery bypass. Postoperatively, the patient develops mediastinitis of the incision. What is the POA indicator for the mediastinitis?

    a. Y

    b. N

    c. U

    d. W

Domain 5 *Management and Leadership*

403. Connie is the education manager for a national coding service company. Once a month she records a webinar for all her coding personnel to review coding updates, answer questions, and provide continuing education. The webinar is recorded so that all personnel have an opportunity to review the material on their own time and at their own convenience. Questions are directed to Connie via email. This is an example of what type of training method?

    a. Asynchronous

    b. Synchronous

    c. Simulation

    d. Classroom-based

404. Which of the following is a risk that must be considered when entering into an outsourcing contract?

    a. Effective resource management

    b. Efficient productivity

    c. Quality problems

    d. Balanced work distribution

405. When implementing health information management training, determining who needs to be trained, who should do the training, how much training is required, and how the training will be accomplished is the responsibility of:

    a. The vendor

    b. Information systems

    c. Health information management

    d. The implementation team

406. Sandy is coder but would like to be a privacy officer one day. Joan, the privacy officer at her hospital, has agreed to help Sandy on her career path. Joan has suggested that Sandy begin to look at master's degree programs and has taken her to a local association meeting where she can begin to network with other privacy officers. This is an example of:

    a. Continuing education

    b. Job rotation

    c. Mentoring

    d. Succession planning

407. A Joint Commission accredited organization must review their formulary annually to ensure a medication's continued:

    a. Safety and dose

    b. Efficiency and efficacy

    c. Efficacy and safety

    d. Dose and efficiency

408. The focus of conflict management is:

    a. Getting personal counseling for the parties involved

    b. Separating the parties involved so that they do not have to work together

    c. Working with the parties involved to find a mutually acceptable solution

    d. Bringing disciplinary action against one party or the other

409. During her new employee orientation, Katie is paired with another coder who shows Katie to her workstation, explains the organization's coding guidelines, takes her to lunch, and explains the online encoder. This orientation is taking place at what level?

    a. Organizational

    b. Departmental

    c. Individual

    d. Administrative

410. Coders at Medical Center Hospital are expected to do a high volume of coding. Their department also includes a clerical support person who handles phone calls, pulls and files records to be coded, and maintains productivity logs. An abstract clerk enters coded data into the health information system. This is an example of _____ work division.

    a. Parallel

    b. Unit

    c. Serial

    d. Serial unit

411. The leader of the coding performance improvement team wants all team members to clearly understand the coding process. What tool could help accomplish this objective?

    a. Flowchart

    b. Force-field analysis

    c. Pareto chart

    d. Scatter diagram

412. What kind of planning addresses long-term needs and sets comprehensive plans of action?

    a. Tactical

    b. Operational

    c. Strategic

    d. Administrative

413. All variances (as related to accounting) should be labeled as either:

    a. Good or bad

    b. Favorable or unfavorable

    c. Positive or negative

    d. Over budget or under budget

414. Monitoring incidents of patients' falls can be used to measure effectiveness of hospital staff. This type of indicator would be considered a(n):

    a. Employee measure

    b. Clinical measure

    c. Human resource measure

    d. Process measure

415. The vision of a health information services department should:

    a. Stand alone as a guiding force for the department

    b. Be developed by the director of the health information services department

    c. Be limited by organizational constraints

    d. Reflect the vision of the organization

416. Capital budgeting differs from operational budgeting in what manner?

    a. It is generally limited to one fiscal year.

    b. It involves high-dollar purchases and multiple-year projects.

    c. It is usually started after completing the operating budget.

    d. It is for purchases other than equipment.

417. In preparation for the implementation of an electronic health record (EHR), Ruth spends most of her training time in the EHR test system clicking through screens and developing workflows. Ruth is most likely what type of sensory learner?

    a. Auditory

    b. Visual

    c. Tactile

    d. Kinesthetic

418. What is the difference between a credential and a license?

    a. Only a credential requires continuing education credits to remain active.

    b. A license is a legal authorization to practice, whereas a credential is a formal agreement.

    c. Only a license requires an applicant to pass a qualifying examination.

    d. There is no difference.

419. Jane's mother is a resident at Apple Valley Nursing Home. Jane is concerned that her mother is developing an ulcer on her hip. Jane has brought concern to the attention of both the director of nursing and the facility administrator with no resolution. Jane contacts the State Department of Health and files a complaint. From this scenario, predict what will occur next at Apple Valley Nursing Home.

    a. Jane will receive a letter thanking her for her concern.

    b. CMS will contact the nursing home administrator by phone.

    c. A health surveyor will visit the nursing home.

    d. The director of nursing will contact CMS.

420. Western States Medical Center consistently sends their HIM staff to AHIMA's component state association annual conference in an effort to provide continuing education and training for these employees. How does this investment in continuing education by Western States Medical Center support their commitment to quality?

    a. By providing a culture of competence through staff development and learning

    b. By allowing employees the opportunity to meet people from other organizations

    c. By providing employees time away from the department

    d. By allowing the organization to spend down its resources

421. Before the on-site survey team leaves the healthcare facility, they meet with the organization's leadership team and provide a report of their findings. This meeting is called:

    a. Closing meeting

    b. Preliminary report

    c. Exit conference

    d. Convening authority

422. What is it called when accrediting bodies such as the Joint Commission, rather than the government, can survey facilities for compliance with the Medicare Conditions of Participation for hospitals?

    a. Deemed status

    b. Judicial decision

    c. Subpoena

    d. Credentialing

423. Generally, substantial performance by one party to a contract will obligate the other party:

    a. To perform their contractual obligations

    b. Not to perform their contractual obligations

    c. To void the contract

    d. To invalidate the contract

424. Annual renewal of fire safety and disaster preparedness are topics that may be addressed best through training known as:

    a. Job rotation

    b. Customer service

    c. In-service education

    d. Pay for performance

425. Which of the following would be considered a discriminatory practice in the employment setting?

    a. Denial of employment based on criminal record.

    b. Screening out an applicant who does not meet the minimum qualifications for the position.

    c. Denial of employment based on religion.

    d. Hiring a person based on vision of the healthcare entity.

426. Which of the following best describes an example of a consumer engagement activity in which HIM professionals might engage?

    a. Coding roundtables

    b. Chargemaster updates

    c. Patient portal training

    d. New employee orientation

427. Which of the following is considered a viable solution to a staff recruitment problem for coding and transcription shortages?

    a. Delegation

    b. Job distribution

    c. Overtime

    d. Telecommuting

428. Under the Americans with Disabilities Act, employees receive protection with respect to their job duties if they are able to perform the necessary functions of a job:

    a. As the job exists

    b. With reasonable accommodations

    c. With changes to the work arrangements

    d. While sharing the job with another employee

429. Which of the following best describes the role of innovation in strategic thinking as compared to other management tools and approaches?

    a. It creates new market opportunities and serves as the driving force behind growth and profitability.

    b. It is an additional function that one learns after mastering other management functions.

    c. It is a replacement for certain leadership functions.

    d. It is the only goal of a strategic leader.

430. At Community Health Services, each budget cycle provides the opportunity to continue or discontinue services based on available resources so that every department or activity must be justified and prioritized annually in order to effectively allocate resources. Community Health uses what type of operational budget?

    a. Activity-based

    b. Fixed

    c. Flexible

    d. Zero-based

431. Disciplinary action:

    a. Should vary based on to whom the employee reports

    b. Should be documented at each step in the process

    c. Should be taken whenever there is a performance problem

    d. Cannot be taken when employees are unionized

432. At the beginning of a recent accreditation visit, the surveyors met with key leaders of the organization. During the meeting, an outline of the schedule was discussed and key interviewees were identified. What is the term for this important accreditation meeting?

    a. Pre-accreditation meeting

    b. Preliminary meeting

    c. Compulsory review

    d. Opening conference

433. Approaches that help an organization to achieve its strategies are called:

    a. Forecasting

    b. Goals

    c. Visioning

    d. Managing

434. The act of granting a healthcare organization or an individual healthcare practitioner permission to provide services of a defined scope in a limited geographical area is called:

    a. Approval

    b. Certification

    c. Accreditation

    d. Licensure

435. Stacy is the nursing manager for the cardiology services at a local hospital. The hospital has recently emphasized a policy requiring all managers to track and report their employees' absences from work. Stacy feels that this requirement is time-consuming and unnecessary. Why would the hospital require their managers to complete this process?

    a. Reports of absences are tabulated and examined for a possible HAI connection.

    b. Reports of absences are used to determine employee satisfaction.

    c. Administration is concerned about the hospital's image in the community.

    d. Administration is attempting to micromanage their clinical services.

436. Which of the following is a characteristic of strategic management?

    a. Shifting the balance of power to the employees

    b. Creating a plan to avoid change within the healthcare entity

    c. A description of specific implementation plans

    d. A plan to improve the healthcare entity's fit with the external world

437. A physician who provides care in a healthcare facility, is not employed by the healthcare entity and therefore not under the direct control or supervision of another, and is personally responsible for his or her negligent acts and carries his or her own professional liability insurance is considered a(n) _____ to the healthcare entity.

    a. Agent

    b. Independent contractor

    c. Supervisor

    d. Vendor

438. An implementation plan is developed to ensure successful execution and includes:

    a. Strategies, goals, and objectives

    b. Vision, mission, and values

    c. External and internal assessments

    d. Timelines, resource needs, and vision

439. Hiring a known and proven employee with an understanding of the organization and improving morale among current employees are both:

    a. Advantages to external recruitment

    b. Disadvantages to external recruitment

    c. Advantages to internal recruitment

    d. Disadvantages to internal recruitment

440. What is the process of finding, soliciting, and attracting new employees called?

    a. Recruitment

    b. Retention

    c. Orientation

    d. Hiring

441. Which of the following statements describes a critical skill for a strategic manager?

    a. Ability to change direction quickly

    b. Ability to deliver results on budget

    c. Ability to envision relationships between trends and opportunities

    d. Ability to design jobs and match peoples' skills to them

442. As part of the CARF accreditation process, reviewers examine policies and procedures, administrative rules and regulations, administrative records, human resource records, and the case records of patients. This process is called:

    a. Performance improvement

    b. Compliance

    c. Document review

    d. Deemed status

443. Which of the following is a characteristic of an organized medical staff as recognized by the Joint Commission?

    a. Peer review activities are optional unless requested by a physician.

    b. Fully licensed physicians are permitted by law to provide patient care services.

    c. Delineation of clinical privileges is not necessary.

    d. The medical staff is not subject to medical staff bylaws or rules, regulations, and policies, and is subject to a professional code of ethics.

444. Which tool is used to determine the most critical areas for training and education for a group of employees?

    a. Performance evaluation

    b. Needs analysis

    c. Orientation assessment

    d. Job specification

445. Which of the following is a statement made by one party to induce another party to enter into a contract?

    a. *Ultra vires*

    b. Warranty

    c. Agreement

    d. Indemnification

446. Use of a variety of content delivery methods to accommodate different types of learners is called:

    a. Blended learning

    b. Programmed learning

    c. Classroom learning

    d. Online learning

447. Which of the following statements is *not* true about a business associate agreement?

    a. It prohibits the business associate from using or disclosing PHI for any purpose other than that described in the contract with the covered entity.

    b. It allows the business associate to maintain PHI indefinitely.

    c. It prohibits the business associate from using or disclosing PHI in any way that would violate the HIPAA Privacy Rule.

    d. It requires the business associate to make available all of its books and records relating to PHI use and disclosure to the Department of Health and Human Services or its agents.

448. A strategy map can be a useful tool because it:

    a. Provides a record of progress toward goals

    b. Provides a visual framework for integrating strategies

    c. Enables others to better understand the vision underlying change

    d. Enables assignment of essential resources to execute the plan

449. Sarah is not clear about why she needs to collect so much data as she performs her HIM job. Sarah's manager explains that the basic premise behind collecting job analysis data is to determine the job requirements and delineate appropriate _____ and _____.

    a. Task frequency; task importance

    b. Position classification; grade level assignments

    c. Management reporting relationships; job specifications

    d. Job crafting; job redesign

450. The HIM director at University Hospital would like to perform a mock survey on the Joint Commission information management standards. The committee that the HIM director should contact is the:

   a. Ethics committee

   b. Medical executive committee

   c. Accreditation committee

   d. Quality management committee

451. Nurse Joan is working in the ICU at University Hospital. She is carrying out Dr. Jones's order for a medication prescribed to one of her patients. She has received the medication and is preparing to administer it to the patient. Upon entering the patient's room, she asks the patient his name and date of birth and compares this information to the label on the medication. Joan then administers the medication to the patient. This scenario is an example of:

   a. Improving communication between hospital staff

   b. Preventing wrong-patient mistakes that can be made in surgery

   c. Using two patient identifiers to verify patient identity

   d. Identifying patient safety risks

452. During the internal assessment component of strategic planning, a successful HIM manager works closely with which of the following groups?

   a. Human resource department at an affiliated clinic information technology department

   b. HIM department at local competitor hospital

   c. Medical staff leadership

   d. Local health department

453. Joe is hired as a floater in a health information department to fill in wherever help is needed. He learns the jobs of several employees. This is an example of:

   a. Outsourcing

   b. Physical training

   c. Cross-training

   d. Performance evaluation

454. Heather and Jim are both coders at Medical Center Hospital. The hospital allows them to set their own hours as long as one of them is in the office between 9:00 a.m. and 3:00 p.m. so they are accessible to physicians. This kind of work arrangement is called:

   a. Telecommuting

   b. Compressed workweek

   c. Outsourcing

   d. Flextime

455. Which of the following would *not* be included in a healthcare entity's strategic profile?

   a. Nature of its threats and opportunities

   b. Nature of its customers or users

   c. Nature of its market segments

   d. Nature of its geographic markets

456. If parties to a contract agree to hold each other harmless for each other's actions or inactions, this is referred to as a(n):

    a. Indemnification

    b. Liability

    c. Offer

    d. Warranty

457. What is the first step in a successful departmental training and development plan?

    a. Designing the curriculum

    b. Selecting the delivery methods

    c. Determining the latest hot topic

    d. Performing a needs analysis

458. The leaders of a healthcare entity are expected to select an entity-wide performance improvement approach and to clearly define how all levels of the entity will monitor and address improvement issues. The Joint Commission requires ongoing data collection that might require possible improvement for which of the following areas?

    a. Operative and other invasive procedures, medication management, and blood and blood product use

    b. Blood and blood product use, medication management, and appointment to the board of directors

    c. Medication management, marketing strategy, and blood use

    d. Operative and other invasive procedures, appointments to the board of directors, and restraint and seclusion use

459. Which of the following is a common outcome of conflict in the workplace?

    a. Increased morale

    b. Increased retention

    c. Feeling of safety

    d. Decreased productivity

460. Which one of the following statements best reflects the current strategic planning environment?

    a. The focus of strategic planning has become narrower in scope.

    b. Because strategic planning is so complex, it requires fairly complex database support.

    c. Strategic plans must project three to five years into the future if they are to be effective.

    d. Because the environment is volatile, strategic planning must be fluid and open to change.

461. Which of the following most likely reflects a breakthrough strategy rather than an operational tactic?

    a. Improving the speed and accuracy of coding

    b. Empowering consumers by providing internet access to test findings and medication summary

    c. Implementing imaging for historical records

    d. Setting up a help desk for physicians in need of technology training

462. The Joint Commission has published a list of abbreviations classified as "Do Not Use" for the purpose of:

    a. Assisting coders to read physician handwriting

    b. Preventing potential medication errors due to misinterpretation

    c. Making terminology consistent in preparation for electronic records

    d. Identifying physicians who are dispensing large quantities of drugs

463. Helen is the HIM department head and has been asked to share a SWOT analysis of her department with her new boss. One aspect of Helen's SWOT analysis indicates that the chart tracking software is over 10 years old and is not compatible with the digital dictation system. In a SWOT analysis, this would be a(n):

    a. Strength

    b. Weakness

    c. Opportunity

    d. Threat

464. Which of the following is an example of a budget used as a controlling tool?

    a. Doing a cost-benefit analysis for a new piece of scanning equipment

    b. Responding to a monthly budget variance report

    c. Preparing a zero-based budget

    d. Creating a cost justification for a budget committee

465. Which of the following are alternate work scheduling techniques?

    a. Compressed workweek, open systems, and job sharing

    b. Flextime, telecommuting, and compressed workweek

    c. Telecommuting, open systems, and flextime

    d. Flextime, outsourcing, compressed workweek

466. The time required to recoup the cost of an investment is called the:

    a. Accounting rate of return

    b. Budget cycle

    c. Payback period

    d. Depreciation

467. Which of the following is true about contracts?

    a. They must be in writing.

    b. They must be express.

    c. They must contain an offer and acceptance.

    d. They must contain a request for proposal.

468. The HIM department at University Hospital is assessing means of remuneration that will impact employee and manager performance. All of the items should be considered when evaluating pay for performance initiatives *except*:

   a. Aggregation of data for assessing pay for performance should be standardized and not require an extensive amount of management time to collect.

   b. Performance appraisals should be designed to account for the nature of job performance.

   c. Human resources does not need to provide training to HIM managers on how to calculate performance appraisal results in relation to pay for performance ratings.

   d. Performance appraisals should have built-in dynamic performance ratings that take into account variable work performance.

469. One of the most common issues that healthcare organizations fail to do well in the strategic process is:

   a. Develop a vision

   b. Develop strategies

   c. Execute the implementation plan

   d. Communicate the plan

470. The percent of antibiotics administered immediately prior to open reduction and internal fixation (ORIF) surgeries or the percent of deliveries accomplished by cesarean section are examples of what type of performance measure?

   a. Outcome measure

   b. Data measure

   c. Process measure

   d. System measure

   Use the following information for questions 471 and 472:

   > At the end of March, the HIM department has a YTD payroll budget of $100,000. The actual YTD amount paid is $95,000 because a coder resigned in February. For the past two months, the position has been filled through outsourcing. Therefore, the actual YTD amount for consulting services is $5,000, although no money was budgeted for consulting services. The reporting threshold for variances is 4 percent. The fiscal year-end is December.

471. What is the best description of the consulting services variance?

   a. Favorable, permanent

   b. Unfavorable, permanent

   c. Favorable, temporary

   d. Unfavorable, temporary

472. Which one of the variances will the HIM director be required to explain?

   a. Only the consulting services variance

   b. Only the payroll variance

   c. Both the payroll and consulting services variances

   d. Neither because the two variances cancel each other out

473. Allowing employees to solve problems within the scope of their job is a characteristic of:

    a. Empowerment

    b. Flexing

    c. Adult learning

    d. Outsourcing

474. The best leader of change is one who:

    a. Can influence behavior

    b. Has the power of position to require change

    c. Offers the best incentives

    d. Serves as a role model

475. The HIM manager was directed by hospital leadership to contract with a vendor to perform the release of information (ROI) function for the organization. Which type of contract will need to be created for this partnership with an ROI vendor?

    a. Temporary

    b. Full service

    c. Emergency

    d. Long term

476. Cory is the project manager for a performance improvement initiative for a large hospital corporation. As part of his duties, he is consistently reviewing the current-status of the project and ensuring that activities are meeting their timeline. If Rob finds that activities are not meeting their timeline, he initiates changes to help the project to get back on track. What phase of project management is Rob performing?

    a. Closure

    b. Monitoring and controlling

    c. Execution

    d. Initiation

477. The HIM department is having an issue with extensive use of sick leave within the department, and quality of work has declined. The HIM manager decides to personally ask each employee in the department what they believe is leading to the problem with extensive use of sick leave. The HIM manager uses this information to create a new sick leave policy in an effort to improve the quality of work performed in the department. What technique is the HIM manager using to address the sick leave and quality of work issue?

    a. Exclusive

    b. Facilitative

    c. Functional

    d. Inclusive

478. The coding supervisor is restructuring staff and rewriting job descriptions to ensure clerical work is no longer required of the coders and physician education is focused with the CDI staff. Which of the following managerial functions best describes this task?

   a. Planning

   b. Organizing

   c. Leading

   d. Controlling

479. The HIM department "ensures secure, complete, and quality documentation of patient care" is an example of a _____.

   a. Vision statement

   b. Values statement

   c. Mission statement

   d. Philosophy statement

480. Which work design tool uses an office layout to visualize the interaction of various work procedures?

   a. Job procedure

   b. Work distribution chart

   c. Workflow process

   d. Movement diagram

481. Which of the following best categorizes the group of adopters who comprise the backbone of the organization, are conventional and deliberate in their decisions, and form a bridge with other adopter categories?

   a. Innovators

   b. Early adopters

   c. Early majority

   d. Late majority

482. The ability to move money from a department's travel budget to the supply budget meets which one of the following characteristics of effective control?

   a. Simplicity

   b. Flexibility

   c. Economy

   d. Focus on exceptions

483. John, HIM department director, recently redesigned the orientation program for two new employees who were assigned to work remotely as coders. After two months, both employees resigned their positions. John is wondering what he can do to prevent this from happening again. Which of the following would you suggest to John?

   a. Spend less time with the employees on their first day and let them work independently

   b. Complete the program in no more than 4 hours

   c. Emphasize that the employee handbook serves as a contract

   d. Review the evaluation forms completed by the employees immediately following the orientation program for ways to improve the program.

484. Larry is creating a recorded webinar to provide updates to coders who work in remote locations. One of the coders is hearing-challenged and requires accommodations so she can benefit from the webinar. Larry's director has told him that according to the Americans with Disabilities Act of 1990, he must provide accommodations for training for any employees who have physical limitations. Which would be a reasonable response by Larry?

    a. Locate a service that can provide captioning or transcription of the audio.

    b. Inform the employee she needs to figure out a solution to this issue, as it is a requirement of her job.

    c. Locate a written source of coding updates as a separate option for this employee and ask the department to pay for it.

    d. Rather than single out one employee, inform all employees they will need to find a source for training on their own prior to the update implementation date.

485. The project manager decided to bring on three additional members to the team a few weeks before the completion deadline to ensure the due date was met. What was the likely result?

    a. The deadline was met right on schedule

    b. The project was completed early

    c. The work plus a few additional tasks were completed by the deadline

    d. The team struggled with multiple delays and missed the deadline

486. What is an unpaid leave of absence initiated by the employer as a strategy for downsizing staff that may result in the employee being called back to work later?

    a. Termination

    b. Suspension

    c. Layoff

    d. Arbitration

487. Michael was so upset that he was required to come in on his approved day off, he wrote a letter of complaint and sent it to the department manager. This is called a(n) _____.

    a. Reprimand

    b. Official warning

    c. Grievance

    d. Amendment

488. The master list of individual accounts maintained by an organization is called the:

    a. Journal

    b. Chargemaster

    c. Budget

    d. General ledger

489. What are the three components of a project plan?

    a. Mission, vision, and goals

    b. Leader, staff, and budget

    c. Scope, budget, and schedule

    d. Goals, resources, and budget

490. In which stage of change, is it postulated that change requires interventions to avoid returning to old ways?

    a. Kubler-Ross Grief Cycle

    b. Kurt Lewin Model of Change Theory

    c. Peter Drucker's Knowledge Worker

    d. Prochaka and DiClemente Stages of Change

491. When a variance in work performance is identified, the next step should be to _____.

    a. Correct the variance

    b. Change the indicator

    c. Analyze the situation

    d. Adjust the budget

492. Which element of the systems model cannot be easily controlled by an organization?

    a. Input

    b. Process

    c. Output

    d. Environment

493. Laggard adopters best serve the function of _____.

    a. Providing a group for downsizing the organization

    b. Providing vision for the organization

    c. Seeking reasons to innovate

    d. Keeping the organization from changing too fast

494. What document outlines the work to be performed by a specific employee or group of employees with the same responsibilities?

    a. Union contract

    b. Policy and Procedure Manual

    c. Job evaluation

    d. Job description

495. Claims paid by third-party payers create transactions that are posted to _____.

    a. Accounts payable and revenue

    b. Accounts receivable and cash

    c. Accounts payable and accounts

    d. Accounts receivable and revenue

496. Project charter is another term for project _____.

    a. Definition

    b. Lessons learned

    c. Work breakdown structure

    d. Planning

497. John is the director of HIM at a large acute-care facility. He is concerned because the coders in his department never seem to be able to keep up with the number of discharges. The chief financial officer (CFO) is questioning the cost of hiring consultants to cover the backlog, because John is in danger of exceeding his consulting budget very soon. John is not sure whether he needs to hire another coder or work more closely with his existing coders to increase productivity. Which of the following activities will be most helpful for John to understand whether his coders are appropriately productive?

    a. Brainstorming

    b. Needs assessment

    c. Benchmarking

    d. Quality improvement

498. Jane is an inpatient coder within the health information management (HIM) department. The HIM coding area has just implemented computer-assisted coding and previously, Jane worked in a facility that had one in place. Jane's boss is relying on Jane to assist her coworkers with transitioning to the new coding product. Jane has a very positive outlook and she encourages her fellow coworkers throughout the day. Jane's behavior is typical of a _____.

    a. Leader

    b. Manager

    c. Subordinate

    d. Follower

499. Which of the following would be considered to be revenue to an outpatient imaging center?

    a. Office supplies

    b. Technicians' salaries

    c. Maintenance agreements for equipment

    d. Radiology procedures

500. A summary of knowledge, skills, abilities, and characteristics required of an individual to perform the job is called the _____.

    a. Orientation plan

    b. Job evaluation

    c. Job specification

    d. Training plan

501. Sheila's lawsuit against her physician-office employer for discrimination due to religious beliefs resulted in a victory for Sheila. She was awarded $500,000 in damages that were intended to send a message that religious discrimination in the workplace would not be tolerated. This payment represents what type of damages paid to an employee?

    a. Compensatory

    b. Retaliatory

    c. Punitive

    d. Claims

502. Which of the following is a critical component of strategic planning?

    a. Identifying budgetary limitations

    b. Selecting a strategic planning consultant

    c. Monitoring the external environment

    d. Setting up committees to define strategies

503. Mary has been taken some classes at the local university on data analysis. She likes her job as a data quality specialist for inpatient coding but she feels like she needs to expand her skills. Mary is looking for _____.

    a. Job enrichment

    b. Job crafting

    c. Job redesign

    d. Job re-evaluation

504. Which method of job evaluation places weight on each of the compensable factors in a job?

    a. Point method

    b. Hay method

    c. Factor comparison method

    d. Job ranking

505. The registration supervisor, Sandy, needs to terminate one of her registration staff. This is the first time she has had to let a staff member go. How should she handle this situation?

    a. Provide notification of termination to the affected employee in writing at least one hour before meeting with the employee to discuss it.

    b. Review all of the issues and problems that led up to the termination decision with the affected employee.

    c. Apologize to the employee for any hurt or anger your termination action will cause them to feel.

    d. Respectfully state her position, provide appropriate severance information, and treat the person with dignity and respect.

506. Betty is the senior transcriptionist at Memorial Hospital. Her supervisor paired Betty with the newest transcriptionist so that Betty might transfer some of her insight and expertise before she retires. This is an example of:

    a. Age discrimination

    b. Bridge employment

    c. Knowledge management

    d. Social identity

507. An electronic health record system implementation was completed over a period of 18 months at a cost of $150,000. During the project, two change orders were approved using the change management process. Change order 113 was for $10,000 and required an additional two months to complete. Change order 123 was for $15,000 and required one additional month to complete. If the project charter established the budget at $95,000 dollars over 16 months, what was the status of the completed project?

    a. Under budget and ahead of schedule

    b. Under budget and late

    c. Over budget and ahead of schedule

    d. Over budget and late

508. During her interview for the position of assistant director of HIM, Jackie spends separate time answering questions with the director of HIM, all of the members of the coding section, and the assistant directors of both the patient financial services (PFS) and information technology (IT) departments. This is an example of what type of interview?

    a. 360-degree interview

    b. Behavioral interview

    c. Structured interview

    d. Unstructured interview

509. During innovations and organizational changes, why is it often said that "things tend to get worse before they get better."

    a. People must learn new skills and doing so may show a drop in performance before they get better at it

    b. People who are laggards slow down the process and things get better after they leave the organization

    c. Performance drop is probably due to so many people involved in planning the change rather than doing their normal work

    d. During change most people already have a negative attitude and it just seems that performance drops

510. Albert is blind and requests that his seeing-eye dog be allowed to accompany him to his job as a transcriptionist at Memorial Hospital. The hospital objects to Albert's request, stating that the dog will aggravate employee allergies and be a general nuisance in the department. Memorial Hospital believes that permitting the dog in the department is an example of:

    a. Bona fide occupational qualification

    b. Reasonable accommodation

    c. Quid pro quo

    d. Undue hardship

511. As the coding manager, Mary has the responsibility of assuring that her coding team meets bill drop deadlines and for reporting her team's weekly productivity statistics to the HIM director. Mary has been given _____ to ensure that her team meets its productivity goals.

    a. Behavioral authority

    b. Scientific authority

    c. Legitimate authority

    d. Humanistic management

512. Which financial statement reflects the extent to which an organization's revenues exceed its expenses?

    a. Balance sheet

    b. Statement of cash flow

    c. Statement of retained earnings

    d. Income statement

513. The HIM director has approval to fill the vacant assistant director position. Even though she knows there are long-standing internal staff who may be interested, she feels it is necessary to hire someone with the RHIA credential. What should she do?

    a. Send the job posting to AHIMA

    b. Only interview RHIAs who apply

    c. Update the job specification section of the job description

    d. Ask HR to screen out internal staff

514. Which of the following is an alternate work schedule option that was made possible by the growth and development of technology?

    a. Compressed workweek

    b. Open systems

    c. Telecommuting

    d. Flextime

515. At Community Memorial Hospital, the coding area has five coders. Each coder is responsible for coding, abstracting, tracking records, answering phones, and maintaining productivity logs. This is an example of _____ work division.

    a. Parallel

    b. Unit

    c. Serial

    d. Serial unit

516. "The decision support department will be known throughout the organization as the epicenter of information" is an example of a _____.

    a. Vision statement

    b. Values statement

    c. Mission statement

    d. Philosophy statement

517. What occurs in Lewin's transition stage of refreezing?

    a. The change becomes status quo

    b. Change and transition continue to be promoted

    c. People are urged to change the organization

    d. Leadership roles become more rigid

518. Daniel, the admission department supervisor, has been receiving complaints about his registration staff. They are making patients late for their appointments because they are so slow and the lines are long. What should Daniel do first to address this problem?

    a. Let staff know that there are complaints

    b. Start registering patients himself when lines get long

    c. Observe the patient registration process

    d. Hire a part-time registrar for busy times

519. The most powerful way for someone to change is through:

    a. Adaptive behavior

    b. Personal motivation

    c. Persuasion

    d. Predicatable rewards/punishment

520. The coding supervisor has been tasked with investigating, choosing, and implementing a computer-assisted coding system within a year and a half. She will need to schedule a multitude of tasks over the next 18 months. What tool do you recommend to her?

    a. Causal loop diagram

    b. Gantt chart

    c. A decision tree

    d. An organization chart

PRACTICE EXAM 1

Domain 1 *Data and Information Governance*

1. Sally is the HIM director at Memorial Hospital and has been asked to compose a record retention policy for the hospital. What should be her first consideration in determining how long paper and electronic records must be retained?

   a. The amount of space allocated for record filing and server set up

   b. The number of paper records currently filed and the number of electronic files added on a daily basis

   c. The most stringent law or regulation in the state, CMS, and accrediting body guidelines and standards

   d. The cost of filing space and equipment

2. A 65-year-old white male was admitted to the hospital on 1/15 complaining of abdominal pain. The attending physician requested an upper GI series and laboratory evaluation of CBC and UA. The x-ray revealed possible cholelithiasis, and the UA showed an increased white blood cell count. The patient was taken to surgery for an exploratory laparoscopy, and a ruptured appendix was discovered. The chief complaint was:

   a. Abdominal pain

   b. Cholelithiasis

   c. Exploratory laparoscopy

   d. Ruptured appendix

3. Mrs. Smith's admitting data indicates that her birth date is March 21, 1948. On the discharge summary, Mrs. Smith's birth date is recorded as July 21, 1948. Which data quality element is missing from Mrs. Smith's health record?

   a. Data accuracy

   b. Data consistency

   c. Data accessibility

   d. Data comprehensiveness

4. The discharge summary must be completed within _____ after discharge for most patients but within _____ for patients transferred to other facilities. Discharge summaries are not always required for patients who were hospitalized for fewer than _____ hours.

   a. 30 days, 48 hours, 24 hours

   b. 14 days, 24 hours, 48 hours

   c. 14 days, 48 hours, 24 hours

   d. 30 days, 24 hours, 48 hours

5. Which of the following is an acceptable means of authenticating a record entry?

   a. The physician's assistant electronically signs for the physician.

   b. The HIM clerk electronically signs using the physician's login.

   c. The charge nurse electronically signs for the physician.

   d. The physician personally signs the entry electronically.

6. A method of documenting nurses' progress notes by recording only abnormal or unusual findings or deviations from the prescribed plan of care is called:

   a. Problem-oriented progress notes

   b. Charting by exception

   c. Consultative notations

   d. Open charting

7. In a long-term care setting, these are problem-oriented frameworks for additional patient assessment based on problem identification items (triggered conditions):

   a. Resident Assessment Protocols (RAPs)

   b. Resident Assessment Instrument (RAI)

   c. Utilization Guidelines (UG)

   d. Minimum Data Sets (MDS)

8. HIM departments may be the hub of identifying, mitigating, and correcting master patient index (MPI) errors. Often that information is not shared with other departments within the healthcare entity. After identifying procedural problems that contribute to the creation of the MPI errors, which department should the MPI manager work with to correct these procedural problems?

   a. Administration

   b. Registration or patient access

   c. Risk management

   d. Radiology and laboratory

9. Alex, an HIM analyst, reviews the record of Patty Eastly, a patient in the facility, to ensure that all documents are complete and signatures are present. This is an example of a:

   a. Closed review

   b. Qualitative review

   c. Concurrent review

   d. Delinquent review

10. What type of information makes it easy for hospitals to compare and combine the contents of multiple patient health records?

    a. Administrative information

    b. Demographic information

    c. Progress notes

    d. Uniform data sets

11. The data elements in a patient's automated laboratory result are examples of:

    a. Unstructured data

    b. Free-text data

    c. Financial data

    d. Structured data

12. Which of the following materials are required elements in an emergency care record?

    a. Patient's instructions at discharge and a complete medical history

    b. Time and means of the patient's arrival, treatment rendered, and instructions at discharge

    c. Time and means of the patient's arrival, patient's complete medical history, and instructions at discharge

    d. Treatment rendered, instructions at discharge, and the patient's complete medical history

13. In assessing the quality of care given to patients with diabetes mellitus, the quality team collects data regarding blood sugar levels on admission and on discharge. These data are called a(n):

    a. Indicator

    b. Measurement

    c. Assessment

    d. Outcome

14. Sue is updating the data dictionary for her organization. In this data dictionary, the data element name is considered which of the following?

    a. Master data

    b. Metadata

    c. Structured data

    d. Unstructured data

15. Which of the following is used by a long-term care facility to gather information about specific health status factors and includes information about specific risk factors in the resident's care?

    a. Case management

    b. Minimum Data Set

    c. Outcomes and assessment information set

    d. Core measure abstracting

16. Dr. Collins admitted John Baker to University Hospital. Blue Cross Insurance will pay John's hospital bill. Upon discharge from the hospital, who owns John's health record?

    a. John

    b. Blue Cross

    c. University Hospital

    d. Dr. Collins

17. Jane Smith emailed her physician, Dr. Ward, to express concern about an abnormal lab value report she received during her last physical exam. Dr. Ward responded to Jane's email by further explaining the lab test and value meanings and then offered various treatment options. How should this email correspondence be handled?

    a. Since this is an email correspondence, the facility has no responsibility to keep it as part of the patient's medical record.

    b. Since this email correspondence relates to communication between a physician and a patient and includes PHI, the facility should include the email in the patient's medical record.

    c. Since this is an email correspondence, it should be kept in a separate social media file within the health information management department.

    d. Since this is an email correspondence, it should be immediately deleted from the server and the physician should be disciplined for discussing PHI related topics via social media.

18. Derek, an HIM technician, reviews each record in the EHR system upon discharge of the patient to ensure that the system correctly assigned all documentation to the correct tab category (for example, all lab reports under the lab tab and x-ray reports under the radiology tab). This system utilizes which format for its patient care record?

    a. Integrated

    b. Practice-oriented

    c. Chronological

    d. Source-oriented

19. A local skilled nursing facility has been working to improve the quality of care it provides to residents. Facility staff have engaged in several PI initiatives recently, and the facility's internal data shows an improvement in quality metrics. The facility administrator is pleased with these findings but is also interested in determining how this facility is performing in contrast to other nearby skilled nursing facilities. Which of the following should the HIM professional use to inform management on how the facility compares to others in the area?

    a. Comparative performance data

    b. Internal infection reporting

    c. Master patient index

    d. Provider performance data

20. According to Joint Commission Accreditation Standards, which document must be placed in the patient's record before a surgical procedure may be performed?

    a. Admission record

    b. Physician's order

    c. Report of history and physical examination

    d. Discharge summary

21. The following data have been collected by the hospital quality committee. What conclusions can be made from the data on the hospital's quality of care between the first and second quarters?

Measure	1st Quarter	2nd Quarter
Medication errors	3.2%	10.4%
Patient falls	4.2%	8.6%
Hospital-acquired infections	1.8%	4.9%
Transfusion reactions	1.4%	2.5%

   a. Quality of care improved between the first and second quarters.

   b. Quality of care is about the same between the first and second quarters.

   c. Quality of care declined between the first and second quarters.

   d. Quality of care should not be judged by these types of measures.

22. The MPI manager has identified a pattern of duplicate health record numbers from the specimen processing area of the hospital. After spending time merging the patient information and correcting the duplicates in the patient information system, the MPI manager needs to notify which department to correct the source system data?

   a. Laboratory

   b. Radiology

   c. Quality management

   d. Registration

23. Borrowing record entries from another source as well as representing or displaying past documentation as current are examples of a potential breach of:

   a. Identification and demographic integrity

   b. Authorship integrity

   c. Statistical integrity

   d. Auditing integrity

24. When defining the legal health record in a healthcare entity, it is best practice to establish a policy statement of the legal health record as well as a:

   a. Case-mix index

   b. Master patient index

   c. Health record matrix

   d. Retention schedule

25. Notes written by physicians and other practitioners as well as dictated and transcribed reports are examples of:

   a. Standardized data

   b. Codified data

   c. Aggregate data

   d. Unstructured clinical information

26. Documentation including the date of action, method of action, description of the disposed record series of numbers or items, service dates, a statement that the records were eliminated in the normal course of business, and the signatures of the individuals supervising and witnessing the process must be included in this:

    a. Authorization

    b. Certificate of destruction

    c. Informed consent

    d. Continuity of care record

27. Decision-making and authority over data-related matters is known as:

    a. Data management

    b. Data administration

    c. Data governance

    d. Data modeling

Domain 2 *Compliance with Access, Use, and Disclosure of Health Information*

28. A professional basketball player from the local team was admitted to your facility for a procedure. During this patient's hospital stay, access logs may need to be checked daily in order to determine:

    a. Whether access by employees is appropriate

    b. If the patient is satisfied with their stay

    c. If it is necessary to order prescriptions for the patient

    d. Whether the care to the patient meets quality standards

29. A patient has the right to request a(n) _____, which describes where the covered entity has disclosed patient information for the past six years outside of treatment, payment, and healthcare operations.

    a. Disclosure list

    b. Designated record set

    c. Amendment of medical record

    d. Accounting of disclosures

30. Why could it be difficult for a healthcare entity to respond to pulling an entire, legal health record together for an authorized request for information?

    a. It can exist in separate and multiple paper-based or electronic systems.

    b. The record is incomplete.

    c. Numerous physicians have not given consent to release the record.

    d. Risk management will not allow the legal health record to be released.

31. Dr. Hansen saw a patient with measles in his office. He directed his office staff to call the local department of health to report this case of measles. The office manager called right away and completed the report as instructed. Which of the following provides the correct analysis of the actions taken by Dr. Hansen's office?

    a. Dr. Hansen's office followed protocol and reported this case of measles correctly.

    b. Dr. Hansen's office did not need to report this case to the local health department.

    c. Dr. Hansen's office should have mailed a letter to the local health department to report this case.

    d. Dr. Hansen's office should have reported the case to the local hospital and not to the health department.

32. What is the implication regarding the confidentiality of incident reports in a legal proceeding when a staff member documents in the health record that an incident report was completed about a specific incident?

    a. There is no impact.

    b. The person making the entry in the health record may not be called as a witness in trial.

    c. The incident report likely becomes discoverable because it is mentioned in a discoverable document.

    d. The incident report cannot be discovered even though it is mentioned in a discoverable document.

33. A hospital receives a valid request from a patient for copies of her medical records. The HIM clerk who is preparing the records removes copies of the patient's records from another hospital where the patient was previously treated. According to HIPAA regulations, was this action correct?

    a. Yes, HIPAA only requires that current records be produced for the patient.

    b. Yes, this is hospital policy over which HIPAA has no control.

    c. No, the records from the previous hospital are considered to be included in the designated record set and should be given to the patient.

    d. No, the records from the previous hospital are not included in the designated record set but should be released anyway.

34. John is the privacy officer at General Hospital and conducts audit log checks as part of his job duties. What does an audit log check for?

    a. Loss of data

    b. Presence of a virus

    c. Successful completion of a backup

    d. Unauthorized access to a system

35. An outpatient laboratory routinely mails the results of health screening exams to its patients. The lab has received numerous complaints from patients who have received another patient's health information. Even though multiple complaints have been received, no change in process has occurred because the error rate is low in comparison to the volume of mail that is processed daily for the lab. How should the Privacy Officer for this healthcare entity respond to this situation?

    a. Determine why the lab results are being sent to incorrect patients and train the laboratory staff on the HIPAA Privacy Rule

    b. Fire the responsible employees

    c. Do nothing, as these types of errors occur in every healthcare entity

    d. Retrain the entire hospital entity because these types of errors could result in a huge fine from the Office of Inspector General

36. Anywhere Hospital's coding staff will be working remotely. The entity wants to ensure that they are complying with the HIPAA Security Rule. What type of network uses a private tunnel through the Internet as a transport medium that will allow the transmission of ePHI to occur between the coder and the facility securely?

    a. Intranet

    b. Local area network

    c. Virtual private network

    d. Wide area network

37. An individual designated as an inpatient coder may have access to an electronic medical record in order to code the record. Under what access security mechanism is the coder allowed access to the system?

    a. Context-based

    b. Role-based

    c. Situation-based

    d. User-based

38. The Security Rule leaves the methods for conducting the security risk analysis to the discretion of the healthcare entity. The first consideration for a healthcare facility should be:

    a. Its own characteristics and environment

    b. The potential threats and vulnerabilities

    c. The level of risk

    d. An assessment of current security measures

39. Sally Mitchell was treated for kidney stones at Graham Hospital last year. She now wants to review her medical record in person. She has requested to review it by herself in a closed room.

    a. Failure to accommodate her wishes will be a violation under the HIPAA Privacy Rule.

    b. Sally owns the information in her record, so she must be granted her request.

    c. Sally's request does not have to be granted because the hospital is responsible for the integrity of the medical record.

    d. Patients should never be given access to their actual medical records.

40. Who has the legal right to refuse treatment?

    1. Juanita who is 98 years old and of sound mind.
    2. Christopher who is 10 years old and of sound mind.
    3. Jane who is 35, incompetent, and did not express her treatment wishes prior to becoming incompetent.
    4. Linda who is 35, incompetent, and created a living will prior to becoming incompetent stating that she did not wish to be kept alive by artificial means.
    5. William who is a 35-year-old born with an intellectual disability and has the mental capacity of a 12-year-old.

    a. 1 and 2

    b. 1 and 3

    c. 1 and 4

    d. 4 and 5

41. Linda Wallace is being admitted to the hospital. She is presented with a Notice of Privacy Practices. In the Notice, it is explained that her PHI will be used and disclosed for treatment, payment, and operations (TPO) purposes. Linda states that she does not want her PHI used for those purposes. Of the options listed here, what is the best course of action?

    a. The hospital must honor her wishes and not use her PHI for TPO.

    b. The hospital may decline to treat Linda because of her refusal.

    c. The hospital is not required to honor her wishes in this situation, as the Notice of Privacy Practices is informational only.

    d. The hospital is not required to honor her wishes for treatment purposes but must honor them for payment and operations purposes.

42. Jack Mitchell, a patient in Ross Hospital, is being treated for heart failure. He has not opted out of the facility directory. Callers who request information about him may be given:

    a. No information due to the highly sensitive nature of his illness

    b. Admission date and location in the facility

    c. General condition and acknowledgment of admission

    d. Location in the facility and diagnosis

43. A data breach occurred in your organization, and after the investigation it was determined that a total of 785 individuals were impacted by the data breach. What must be completed within 60 days of learning about the data breach?

    a. Update the notice of privacy practices and send to all patients

    b. Report the incident to the individuals impacted, local media, and the Department of Health and Human Services

    c. Conduct privacy training for members of the organization

    d. Document a note mentioning the data breach in each of the patients' charts and tell the local media

44. The "custodian of health records" refers to the individual within a healthcare entity who is responsible for which of the following actions?

    a. Determining alternative treatment for the patient

    b. Preparing physicians to testify

    c. Testifying to the authenticity of records

    d. Testifying regarding the care of the patient

45. Dr. Smith, a member of the medical staff, asks to see the medical records of his adult daughter who was hospitalized in your institution for a tonsillectomy at age 16. The daughter is now 25. Dr. Jones was the patient's physician. Of the options listed here, what is the best course of action?

    a. Allow Dr. Smith to see the records because he was the daughter's guardian at the time of the tonsillectomy.

    b. Call the hospital administrator for authorization to release the record to Dr. Smith since he is on the medical staff.

    c. Inform Dr. Smith that he cannot access his daughter's health record without her signed authorization allowing him access to the record.

    d. Refer Dr. Smith to Dr. Jones and release the record if Dr. Jones agrees.

46. St. Joseph's Hospital has a psychiatric service on the sixth floor. A 31-year-old male came to the HIM department and requested to see a copy of his health record. He told the clerk he was a patient of Dr. Schmidt, a psychiatrist, and had been on the sixth floor of St. Joseph's for the last two months. These records are not psychotherapy notes. The best course of action for you to take as the HIM director is:

    a. Prohibit the patient from accessing his record as it contains psychiatric diagnoses that may greatly upset him.

    b. Allow the patient to access his record.

    c. Allow the patient to access his record if, after contacting his physician, his physician does not feel it will be harmful to the patient.

    d. Deny access because HIPAA prevents patients from reviewing their psychiatric records.

47. You are a member of the hospital's Health Information Management Committee. The committee has created a HIPAA-compliant authorization form. Which of the following items does the Privacy Rule require for the form?

    a. Signature of the patient's attending physician

    b. Identification of the patient's next of kin

    c. Identification of the person or entity authorized to receive PHI

    d. Patient's insurance information

48. Protected health information that is maintained in a designated record set can be accessed by the patient or other authorized party upon request. Covered entities must respond to requests within what timeframe after receipt of the request?

    a. 15 days

    b. 30 days

    c. 60 days

    d. 90 days

49. A hospital health information department receives a subpoena duces tecum for records of a former patient. When the health record professional goes to retrieve the patient's medical records, it is discovered that the records being subpoenaed have been purged in accordance with the state retention laws. In this situation, how should the HIM department respond to the subpoena?

    a. Inform defense and plaintiff lawyers that the records no longer exist

    b. Submit a certification of destruction in response to the subpoena

    c. Refuse the subpoena since no records exist

    d. Contact the clerk of the court and explain the situation

50. An HIM professional violates privacy protection under the HIPAA Privacy Rule when he or she releases _____ without specific authorization from the patient(s) or patient representative(s).

    a. A list of newborns to the local newspaper for publication in the birth announcements section

    b. Data about cancer patients to the state health department cancer surveillance program

    c. Birth information to the country registrar

    d. Information about patients with sexually transmitted infections to the county health department

51. What is the implication regarding the confidentiality of incident reports in a legal proceeding when a staff member documents in the health record that an incident report was completed about a specific incident?

    a. There is no impact.

    b. The person making the entry in the health record may not be called as a witness in trial.

    c. The incident report likely becomes discoverable because it is mentioned in a discoverable document.

    d. The incident report cannot be discovered even though it is mentioned in a discoverable document.

52. The use of electronic information and telecommunications technologies to support long-distance clinical healthcare, patient and professional health-related education, public health, and health administration is called:

    a. Secure messaging

    b. Consumer informatics

    c. Personalized medicine

    d. Telehealth

53. In order for health information exchange (HIE) participants to search for health records on each of the other systems using patient indexing and identification software, the systems must be linked by a(n):

    a. Primary key interface (PKI)

    b. Application programming interface (API)

    c. Continuity of care record (CCR)

    d. Record locator service (RLS)

54. Which of the following is the unique identifier in the relational database patient table?

Patient Table			
Patient #	**Patient Last Name**	**Patient First Name**	**Date of Birth**
021234	Smith	Donna	03/21/1944
022366	Jones	Donna	04/09/1960
034457	Smith	Mary	08/21/1977

    a. Patient last name

    b. Patient last and first name

    c. Patient date of birth

    d. Patient number

55. In a relational database, which of the following is an example of a many-to-many relationship?

    a. Patients to hospital admissions

    b. Patients to consulting physicians

    c. Patients to hospital health records

    d. Primary care physician to patients

56. A possible justification for building an information system in-house rather than purchasing one from a vendor is that:

    a. It is cheaper to buy than to build

    b. The facility has development teams they do not want to give up

    c. Integration of systems will be easier

    d. Vendor products are not comprehensive enough

57. What is the formatting problem in the following table?

Medical Center Hospital Admission Types		
Elective	2,843	62.4
Emergency admission	942	37.6
Total	3,785	100.0

    a. The variable names are missing

    b. The title of the table is missing

    c. The column headings are missing

    d. The column totals are inaccurate

58. Community Memorial Hospital had 25 inpatient deaths, including newborns, during the month of June. The hospital had a total of 500 discharges for the same period, including deaths of adults, children, and newborns. The hospital's gross death rate for the month of June was:

    a. 0.05%

    b. 2%

    c. 5%

    d. 20%

59. In which of the following phases of systems selection and implementation would the process of running a mock query to assess the functionality of a database be performed?

    a. Initial study

    b. Design

    c. Testing

    d. Operation

60. In the data warehouse, the patient's last name and first name are entered into separate fields. This is an example of what?

    a. Query

    b. Normalization

    c. Key field

    d. Slicing and dicing

61. A physician is interested in conducting research on herniated intervertebral disc disease. She wants to compare the success of conservative medical care versus surgical intervention. The best source of this information is the:

    a. Disease index

    b. Operative index

    c. Master patient index

    d. Trauma registry

62. The health information services department at Medical Center Hospital has identified problems with its work processes. Too much time is spent on unimportant tasks, there is duplication of effort, and task assignment is uneven in quality and volume among employees. What should the manager do?

    a. The manager should have each employee complete a serial work request.

    b. The manager should have each employee complete a work distribution chart.

    c. The manager should have the employees complete a use case analysis.

    d. The manager should develop a flow process chart.

63. By querying the healthcare entity data, you find that patients admitted on a weekend have a mean length of stay that is 1.3 days longer than patients who are admitted Monday through Friday. This method of finding information is called:

    a. Structuring query language

    b. Data mining

    c. Multidimensional data structuring

    d. Satisficing

64. A health information professional is preparing statistical information about the third-party payers that reimburse care in the facility. She finds the following information: Medicare reimburses 46 percent; Medicaid reimburses 13 percent; Blue Cross reimburses 21 percent; workers' compensation reimburses 1 percent; commercial plans reimburse 15 percent; and other payers or self-payers reimburse 4 percent. What is the best graphic tool to use to display this data?

    a. Histogram

    b. Pie chart

    c. Line graph

    d. Table

65. During an influenza outbreak, a nursing home reports 25 new cases of influenza in a given month. These 25 cases represent 30 percent of the nursing home's population. This rate represents the:

    a. Distribution

    b. Frequency

    c. Incidence

    d. Prevalence

66. When a physician office acquires a new EHR in place of its old EHR, the old EHR data will require:

    a. Chart conversion

    b. Chart transition

    c. Data conversion

    d. Data processing

67. Using the admission criteria provided, determine if the following patient meets the severity of illness and intensity of service criteria for admission.

Severity of Illness	Intensity of Service
Persistent fever	Inpatient-approved surgery/procedure within 24 hours of admission
Active bleeding	Intravenous medications or fluid replacement
Wound dehiscence	Vital signs every 2 hours or more often

Sue presents with vaginal bleeding. An ultrasound showed a missed abortion so she is being admitted to the outpatient surgery suite for a D&C.

a. The patient does not meet both severity of illness and intensity of service criteria.

b. The patient does meet both severity of illness and intensity of service criteria.

c. The patient meets intensity of service criteria but not severity of illness.

d. The patient meets severity of illness criteria but not intensity of service.

68. The user needs a list of all of the patients that were diagnosed with a cerebral infarction or a cerebral hemorrhage. What type of search would be used in this situation?

a. Structured query language

b. Wildcard search

c. Truncation

d. Boolean search

69. A hospital is conducting an analysis of its existing health information systems and is looking at potential areas that need attention. This step is typically referred to as:

a. Identify needs

b. Monitor results

c. Record feedback

d. Specify requirements

70. Community Memorial Hospital discharged nine patients on April 1. The length of stay for each patient is shown in the following table. The average length of stay for these nine patients was:

Patient	Number of Days
A	1
B	5
C	3
D	3
E	8
F	8
G	8
H	9
I	9

a. 5 days

b. 6 days

c. 8 days

d. 9 days

71. The department of surgery has acquired an analytics engine to enable it to provide predictive information at the point of care via the EHR. However, the department is struggling to get physicians to use the functionality because it does not have support staff to program or train users. This situation refers to the fact that the project plan did not illustrate:

    a. Conflicts

    b. Dependencies

    c. Environmental issues

    d. Policy decisions

72. This Health Information Exchange (HIE) consent model requires the patient to give their consent for the inclusion of their data in the HIE.

    a. Opt-in

    b. Opt-out

    c. Automatic consent

    d. No-consent

73. Given the information here, the case-mix index would be:

MS-DRG	MDC	Type	MS-DRG Title	Weight	Discharges	Geometric Mean	Arithmetic Mean
191	04	MED	Chronic obstructive pulmonary disease w CC	0.8642	10	2.7	3.3
192	04	MED	Chronic obstructive pulmonary disease w/o CC/MCC	0.6521	20	2.2	2.6
193	04	MED	Simple pneumonia & pleurisy w MCC	1.2987	10	4.0	5.1
194	04	MED	Simple pneumonia & pleurisy w CC	0.8402	20	2.9	3.6
195	04	MED	Simple pneumonia & pleurisy w/o CC/MCC	0.6418	10	2.3	2.8

    a. 0.09

    b. 0.6521

    c. 0.8270

    d. 82.70

74. A super user of health IT has complained to her supervisor that she is being asked by a physician to perform his data entry. What should the super user's role be?

    a. Aid others in using a new system during go-live and getting to adoption

    b. Serve as a scribe for physicians who are new to data entry

    c. Train users to learn how to use the system prior to go-live

    d. Troubleshoot issues with the system that did not come to light during testing

75. Which of the following do HIE participants use to search for health records on other healthcare organization systems using patient indexing and identification software?

    a. Admit, discharge, transfer

    b. Advance patient identifier

    c. Continuity of care document

    d. Record locator service

76. Which of the following would likely be recorded on an information systems issues log?

    a. Alan is present every day there is a system test.

    b. Betty reported receiving 25 erroneous e-mail messages.

    c. Dr. Brown effectively uses e-prescribing.

    d. John requested a supply of tamperproof paper for his office.

77. A physician is concerned that the data patients enter into an EHR is not as reliable as data entered by another provider. What function serves to distinguish the source of data in an EHR?

    a. Data dictionary

    b. Data provenance

    c. Data quality

    d. Data registry

78. A coding manager wants to display the patient types that have the most coding errors in relationship to coder years of service. The desire of the coding manager is to display how coder years of service is responsible for coding errors. The type of graph or chart best suited for this is a:

    a. Bar graph

    b. Pareto chart

    c. Pie chart

    d. Line graph

79. The best way to ensure that elements of a health information system work together is to:

    a. Adopt all components from a single vendor

    b. Ensure standards are applied to software development that support interoperability

    c. Use an application service provider that supports all vendors

    d. Verify that a vendor applies a systems' view to its product development

80. Using the information in these partial attribute lists for the PATIENT, VISIT, and CLINIC columns in a relational database, the attribute PATIENT_MRN is listed in both the PATIENT Entity Attributes and the VISIT Entity Attributes, and CLINIC_ID is listed in both the VISIT Entity Attributes and the CLINIC Entity Attributes. What does the attribute PATIENT_MRN represent?

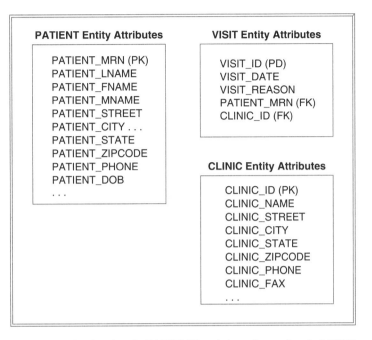

a. It is the foreign key in PATIENT and the primary key in VISIT.

b. It is the primary key in PATIENT and the foreign key in VISIT.s

c. It is the primary key in both PATIENT and VISIT.

d. It is the foreign key in both PATIENT and VISIT.

81. A hospital is conducting an analysis of its existing health information systems and is looking at potential areas that need attention. This step in the systems development life cycle is typically referred to as _____.

a. Identify needs

b. Monitor results

c. Record feedback

d. Specify requirements

82. Patients at the new cardiac clinic at ABC Hospital are given smart watches with special sensors to monitor their blood pressure, heart rate, and rhythm in ECG format to identify any abnormalities during their daily routine. The information generated from these smart devices is considered a:

a. Source system

b. Interoperability system

c. Virtual system

d. Hybrid system

83. One of the older cardiologists expressed dissatisfaction with using an EHR, stating that he does not understand why it's necessary. Sandy, as the EHR Clinical Coordinator, talks about his work as the first physician at ABC Hospital to use computerized technology for cardiac patients, and how cardiac diagnosis outcomes improved. She relates to him that the EHR will have the same impact and that the best reason to implement an EHR is to:

    a. Determine the cost of care

    b. Improve patient care

    c. Eliminate medical errors

    d. Meet Joint Commission mandate for the EHR

84. Dr. Wilson asks you, the EHR Manager, to explain the difference between an alert and a reminder. You explain that reminders are typically used for things that can be scheduled or that occur on a regular basis. An example of a reminder that would be given to Dr. Wilson would be:

    a. Use of anticoagulant is contraindicated

    b. Patient is due for MMR immunization

    c. Patient is allergic to sulfa drugs

    d. Drug does not come in this format

85. Using the information in these partial attribute lists for the PATIENT, VISIT, and CLINIC columns in a relational database, the attribute PATIENT_MRN is listed in both the PATIENT Entity Attributes and the VISIT Entity Attributes, and CLINIC_ID is listed in both the VISIT Entity Attributes and the CLINIC Entity Attributes. What does the attribute CLINIC_ID represent?

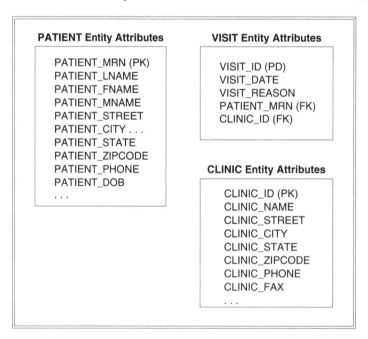

    a. It is the foreign key in CLINIC and the primary key in VISIT.

    b. It is the primary key in CLINIC and the foreign key in VISIT.

    c. It is the primary key in both CLINIC and VISIT.

    d. It is the foreign key in both CLINIC and VISIT.

Revenue Cycle Management

86. A 45-year-old woman is admitted for blood loss anemia due to dysfunctional uterine bleeding.

D25.9	Leiomyoma of uterus, unspecified
D50.0	Iron deficiency anemia secondary to blood loss (chronic)
D62	Acute posthemorrhagic anemia
N93.8	Other specified abnormal uterine and vaginal bleeding

   a. D50.0, N93.8

   b. D62, N93.8

   c. N93.8, D50.0

   d. D50.0, D25.9

87. A coder notes that the patient is taking prescribed Haldol. The final diagnoses on the progress notes include diabetes mellitus, acute pharyngitis, and malnutrition. What condition might the coder suspect the patient has that the physician should be queried to confirm?

   a. Insomnia

   b. Hypertension

   c. Mental or behavioral problems

   d. Rheumatoid arthritis

88. A patient has a malunion of an intertrochanteric fracture of the right hip that is treated with a proximal femoral osteotomy by incision. What is the correct ICD-10-PCS code for this procedure?

Section	Body System	Root Operation	Body Part	Approach	Device	Qualifier
Medical and Surgical	Lower Bones	Excision	Upper Femur, Right	Open	No Device	No Qualifier
0	Q	B	6	0	Z	Z

Section	Body System	Root Operation	Body Part	Approach	Device	Qualifier
Medical and Surgical	Lower Bones	Division	Upper Femur, Right	Open	No Device	No Qualifier
0	Q	8	6	0	Z	Z

Section	Body System	Root Operation	Body Part	Approach	Device	Qualifier
Medical and Surgical	Lower Joints	Excision	Hip Joint, Right	Open	No Device	No Qualifier
0	S	B	9	0	Z	Z

Section	Body System	Root Operation	Body Part	Approach	Device	Qualifier
Medical and Surgical	Lower Joints	Release	Hip Joint, Right	Open	No Device	No Qualifier
0	S	N	9	0	Z	Z

   a. 0QB60ZZ

   b. 0Q860ZZ

   c. 0SB90ZZ

   d. 0SN90ZZ

89. Medical identity thefts are situations in which the following occurs:

    a. When health information on the wrong patient is put in the incorrect record

    b. When financial information is used to purchase nonmedical items

    c. When demographic and financial information is used to acquire medical services

    d. When demographic information is used to purchase nonmedical items

90. A patient is admitted with right diabetic cataract and extracapsular cataract extraction with simultaneous insertion of intraocular lens.

    | E11.36 | Type 2 diabetes mellitus with diabetic cataract |
    | E11.9 | Type 2 diabetes mellitus without complications |
    | H25.9 | Unspecified age-related cataract |
    | H26.9 | Unspecified cataract |

Section	Body System	Root Operation	Body Part	Approach	Device	Qualifier
Medical and Surgical	Eye System	Extraction	Lens, Right	Percutaneous	No Device	No Qualifier
0	8	D	J	3	Z	Z

Section	Body System	Root Operation	Body Part	Approach	Device	Qualifier
Medical and Surgical	Eye System	Replacement	Lens, Right	Percutaneous	Synthetic Substitute	No Qualifier
0	8	R	J	3	J	Z

    a. H25.9, E11.36, 08DJ3ZZ

    b. E11.36, 08RJ3JZ

    c. E11.9, E11.36, H26.9, 08DJ3ZZ

    d. E25.9, E11.9, 08RJ3JZ

91. The practice of using a code that results in a higher payment to the provider than the code that actually reflects the service or item provided is known as:

    a. Unbundling

    b. Billing for services not provided

    c. Medically unnecessary services

    d. Upcoding

92. You are the coding supervisor and you are doing an audit of outpatient coding. Robert Thompson was seen in the outpatient department with a chronic cough, and the record states "rule out lung cancer." What should have been coded as the patient's diagnosis?

    a. Chronic cough

    b. Observation and evaluation without need for further medical care

    c. Diagnosis of unknown etiology

    d. Lung cancer

93. Using the following custom revenue production report, which coding error may be demonstrated in the report?

Revenue Production Report—Small Multispecialty Group Month: January				
Code	Quantity	Fee	Projected Revenue	Actual Insurance Revenue
99202	3	$75	$225	$164.10
99203	4	$90	$360	$267.94
99204	0	$120	$0	$0.00
99205	0	$150	$0	$0.00
99211	703	$28	$19,684	$14,988.32
99212	489	$47	$22,983	$18,092.65
99213	1853	$63	$116,739	$92,890.38
99214	41	$89	$3,649	$2,799.11
99215	7	$135	$945	$722.87
99242	9	$125	$1,125	$156.23
99243	27	$150	$4,050	$610.45
99244	10	$175	$1,750	$124.32
99245	1	$200	$200	$53.10

a. Clustering

b. Unbundling

c. Missed charges

d. Overcoding

94. Jim was admitted for hip replacement surgery, and during his procedure he was administered blood products. Postoperatively, Jim developed a rash and fever. The presence of these symptoms will be investigated by the hospital as a possible:

a. Blood verification

b. Core measure

c. Comorbidity

d. Transfusion reaction

95. Community Hospital has received a large number of claims denials for CT scans that were provided to patients. After review of the denied claims, the hospital has determined that clinical indications for the CT scan were not present. For which of the following reasons were these claims denied for payment?

a. Patient preferences were ignored.

b. These scans did not meet medical necessity.

c. No order was present in the record for the scans.

d. Best practices for billing were not used.

96. The health plan reimburses Dr. Tan $15 per patient per month. In January, Dr. Tan saw 300 patients, so he received $4,500 from the health plan. What method is the health plan using to reimburse Dr. Tan?

    a. Traditional retrospective

    b. Capitated rate

    c. Relative value

    d. Discounted fee schedule

97. Jennifer, the HIM Assistant Director, is establishing her yearly calendar with all the dates for standing monthly committee meetings, weekly production reports, daily census tracking graphs, quarterly payroll accounts, etc. Identify the frequency Jennifer would schedule the chargemaster software updates.

    a. Annually

    b. Quarterly

    c. Monthly

    d. Weekly

98. The technology commonly utilized for automated claims processing (sending bills directly to third-party payers) is:

    a. Optical character recognition

    b. Bar coding

    c. Neural networks

    d. Electronic data interchange

99. A physician performed a total abdominal hysterectomy with bilateral salpingo-oophorectomy on his patient at Community Hospital. His office billed the following:

    | 58150 | Total abdominal hysterectomy (corpus and cervix), with or without removal of tube(s), with or without removal of ovary(s) |
    | 58720 | Salpingo-oophorectomy, complete or partial, unilateral or bilateral (separate procedure) |

    Why was this claim rejected?

    a. Billed hysterectomy with wrong CPT code

    b. Not a covered procedure

    c. Unbundled procedures

    d. Covered procedure but insurance company requires additional information

100. A patient saw a neurosurgeon for treatment of a nerve that was severed in an industrial accident. The patient worked for Basic Manufacturing Company where the industrial accident occurred. Basic Manufacturing carried workers' compensation insurance. The workers' compensation insurance paid the neurosurgeon fees. Which entity is the "third party"?

    a. Patient

    b. Neurosurgeon

    c. Basic Manufacturing Company

    d. Workers' compensation insurance

101. Alfred is tracking the amount of time it takes for physicians to respond to coding queries. He has found that these delays have caused a 30% increase in turn-around time for submitting the bills for reimbursement. The system would assist him and the coders to have the necessary information to make timely coding assignment.

    a. CDM

    b. CPT

    c. CDI

    d. RCM

102. A physician query may not be appropriate in which of the following instances?

    a. Diagnosis of viral pneumonia noted in the progress notes and sputum cultures showing *Haemophilus influenzae*

    b. Discharge summary indicates chronic renal failure but the progress notes document acute renal failure throughout the stay

    c. Acute respiratory failure in a patient whose lab report findings appear to not support this diagnosis

    d. Diagnosis of chest pain and abnormal cardiac enzymes indicative of an AMI

103. The financial manager of the physician group practice explained that the healthcare insurance company would be reimbursing the practice for its treatment of the exacerbation of congestive heart failure that Mrs. Zale experienced. The exacerbation, treatment, and resolution covered approximately five weeks. The payment covered all the services that Mrs. Zale incurred during the period. What method of reimbursement was the physician group practice receiving?

    a. Traditional

    b. Episode-of-care

    c. Per diem

    d. Fee-for-service

104. Allowing patterns of retrospective documentation, hiding or ignoring negative quality review outcomes, and hiding incomplete health records from accreditation surveyors are unethical behaviors according to which of the following Code of Ethics principles?

    a. Advocate and uphold the right to privacy

    b. Respect the inherent dignity and worth of every person

    c. Represent the profession accurately to the public

    d. Put service before self-interest

105. Community Hospital is trying to improve its compliance with Medicare quality reporting requirements and, in turn, its reimbursement from Medicare's Hospital Value-Based Purchasing Program. The hospital has added a _____ to assist in educating medical staff members on documentation needed for accurate billing.

    a. Physician advisor

    b. Compliance officer

    c. Chargemaster coordinator

    d. Data monitor

106. The following table is an example of an:

Patient/Service	Service Date(s)	(A) Total Charge	(B) Not Payable by Plan		Plan Paid Amount	
White, Jane						
Office Visit	02/17/201X	$56.00	$10.00	CP*	$46.00	100%
X-Ray	02/17/201X	$268.00	$250.00			
$3.60	DD* CI*	$14.40	80%			
Lab	02/17/201X	$20.00	$15.00	CP*	$5.00	100%
Total						
*CI: Coinsurance; CP: Copayment; DD: Deductible						

a. Insurance coverage advanced notice service waiver

b. Explanation of benefits

c. Insurance claim form

d. Encounter form

107. Which of the following healthcare entities' mission is to reduce Medicare improper payments through detection and collection of overpayments, identification of underpayments, and implementation of actions that will prevent future improper payments?

a. Accountable care entity

b. Managed care entity

c. Revenue reduction contractor

d. Recovery audit contractor

108. The coding manager at Community Hospital is seeing an increased number of physicians failing to document the cause and effect of diabetes and its manifestations. Which of the following will provide the most comprehensive solution to handle this documentation issue?

a. Have coders continue to query the attending physician for this documentation.

b. Present this information at the next medical staff meeting to inform physicians on documentation standards and guidelines.

c. Do nothing because coding compliance guidelines do not allow any action.

d. Place all offending physicians on suspension if the documentation issues continue.

109. A patient arrived via ambulance to the emergency department following a motor vehicle accident. The patient sustained a fracture of the ankle, a 3.0-cm superficial laceration of the left arm, a 5.0-cm laceration of the scalp with exposure of the fascia, and a concussion. The patient received the following procedures: x-ray of the ankle that showed a bimalleolar ankle fracture requiring closed manipulative reduction, simple suturing of the arm laceration, and layer closure of the scalp. Provide CPT codes for the procedures performed in the emergency department for the facility bill.

12002	Simple repair of superficial wounds of scalp, neck, axillae, external genitalia, trunk and/or extremities (including hands and feet); 2.6 cm to 7.5 cm
12004	Simple repair of superficial wounds of scalp, neck, axillae, external genitalia, trunk and/or extremities (including hands and feet); 7.6 cm to 12.5 cm
12032	Repair, intermediate, wounds of scalp, axillae, trunk and/or extremities (excluding hands and feet); 2.6 cm to 7.5 cm
27810	Closed treatment of bimalleolar ankle fracture (e.g., lateral and medial malleoli, or lateral and posterior malleoli, or medial and posterior malleoli); with manipulation
27818	Closed treatment of trimalleolar ankle fracture; with manipulation
−58	Staged or related procedure or service by the same physician or other qualified health care professional during the postoperative period
−59	Distinct procedural service

a. 27810, 12032

b. 27818, 12004, 12032-58

c. 27810, 12032, 12002-59

d. 27810, 12004

110. What qualifier is used with the root operation excision, extraction, or drainage that are considered diagnostic?

a. D

b. J

c. X

d. Z

111. In conducting a qualitative review, the clinical documentation specialist sees that the nursing staff has documented the patient's skin integrity on admission to support the presence of a stage I pressure ulcer. However, the physician's documentation is unclear as to whether this condition was present on admission. How should the clinical documentation specialist proceed?

a. Note the condition as present on admission

b. Query the physician to determine if the condition was present on admission

c. Note the condition as unknown on admission

d. Note the condition as not present on admission

112. Phil White had coronary artery bypass graft surgery. Unfortunately, during the surgery, Phil suffered a severe stroke. Phil's recovery included several settings in the continuum of care: acute-care hospital, physician office, rehabilitation center, and home health agency. This initial service and subsequent recovery lasted 10 months. As a member of a managed care organization in an integrated delivery system, how should Phil expect that his healthcare billing will be handled?

   a. Bills for each service from each physician, each facility, and each other healthcare provider from every encounter

   b. Bills for each service from each physician, each facility, and each other healthcare provider at the end of the 10-month period

   c. Consolidated billing for each encounter that includes the bills from all the physicians, facilities, and other healthcare providers involved in the encounter

   d. One fixed amount for the entire episode that is divided among all the physicians, facilities, and other healthcare providers

113. The coding supervisor has compiled a report on the number of coding errors made each day by the coding staff. The report data show that Tim makes an average of six errors per day, Jane makes an average of five errors per day, and Bob and Susan each make an average of two errors per day. Given this information, what action should the coding supervisor take?

   a. Counsel Tim and Jane because they have the highest error rates

   b. Encourage Tim and Jane to get additional training

   c. Provide Bob and Susan with incentive pay for low coding error rates

   d. Take no action since not enough information is given to make a judgment

114. Once all data has been posted to patient's account, the claim can be reviewed for accuracy and completeness. Many facilities have an internal auditing system that runs each claim through a set of edits. This internal auditing system is known as a:

   a. Chargemaster

   b. Superbill

   c. Scrubber

   d. Grouper

115. Which of the following terms is used to describe the requirement of the healthcare provider to obtain permission from the health insurer prior to providing service to the patient?

   a. Preauthorization

   b. Advance beneficiary notification

   c. Point of care collection

   d. Local coverage determination

116. Joan is educating the physicians in her hospital about the Medicare Hospital Value-Based Purchasing (VBP) Program. As part of this education she explains to her audience that the HCAHPS survey results are a part of the _____ domain in the Medicare VBP program.

    a. Safety

    b. Clinical Care

    c. Efficiency and Cost Reduction

    d. Person/Community Engagement

117. A series of terms in parentheses that sometimes directly follow main terms in the alphabetic index to diseases ICD-10-CM coding system is called:

    a. exclude note

    b. subterm

    c. nonessential modifier

    d. essential modifier

Domain 5 *Management and Leadership*

118. Sam is the new HIM supervisor. His first assignment is to evaluate the efficiency and effectiveness of his work unit. He has met with the unit's customers to determine their expectations and met with his staff to understand their roles. In setting up systems to measure work performance, it is critical for Sam to establish:

    a. Proper ergonomics

    b. Standards

    c. Action plans

    d. Work distribution charts

119. Pressed for time, Sara hired a new release of information clerk without doing a reference check. When the new clerk committed a violation of patient confidentiality, it came to light that she had committed similar violations at her previous place of employment. By not checking the clerk's references, Sara has opened the hospital to charge of:

    a. Discrimination

    b. Harassment

    c. Negligent hiring

    d. Overcompensation

120. The slightly higher wage paid to an employee who works a less desirable shift is called a:

    a. Shift rotation

    b. Performance incentive

    c. Shift differential

    d. Work distribution ladder

121. Which of the following best differentiates the role of strategic management and strategic thinking as compared to other management tools and approaches?

    a. A component of each of the major functions of management

    b. An additional function that one learns after mastering other management functions

    c. A replacement for certain management functions

    d. A role for senior managers and board of trustees

122. Jan, the new release of information manager, is participating in management orientation for the healthcare organization. One section of orientation thoroughly reviews the tools and practices for setting sustainable performance goals for employees, how to monitor employee progress toward job performance goals, and ways to provide feedback to employees regarding job performance. This section of orientation is called:

    a. Performance management

    b. Situational strength

    c. Critical incident method

    d. Benchmarking

123. Which Joint Commission survey methodology involves an evaluation that follows the hospital experiences of current patients?

    a. Priority focus review

    b. Periodic performance review

    c. Tracer methodology

    d. Performance improvement

124. Employees covered by the provisions of the Fair Labor Standards Act (FLSA) are called _____ employees.

    a. Waged

    b. Salaried

    c. Exempt

    d. Nonexempt

125. A technique for measuring healthcare entity performance across the four perspectives of customer, financial, internal processes, and learning and growth is called:

    a. Strategy map

    b. Process innovations

    c. Balanced scorecard methodology

    d. SWOT analysis

126. As part of his role at the local hospital, Jake is reviewing Joint Commission standards to ensure that the organization is meeting the accreditation requirements. As part of the review, Jake is looking at a specific set of standards that are primarily focused on documentation. Some of the standard requirements include care provided, procedures that were done on the patient, and the progress of the patient. Based on this scenario, which set of Joint Commission standards is Jake reviewing?

    a. Information management standards

    b. Record of care standards

    c. Performance improvement standards

    d. Information resource standards

127. During new employee orientation, Elise, the assistant director of human resources, oversees diversity and sexual harassment training. This orientation is taking place at what level?

    a. Organizational

    b. Departmental

    c. Individual

    d. Administrative

128. The HIM department records copy fees as revenue. For the year the budgeted fees were $25,000 and the actual fees received are $23,000. The director may be asked to explain a(n):

    a. Favorable variance of $2,000

    b. Unfavorable variance of $2,000

    c. Favorable variance of $23,000

    d. Unfavorable variance of $23,000

129. Joe Smith, RHIA, works for an outsourcing company as interim health information department director in a large hospital. By the terms of the contract, the hospital pays the company for Joe's services based on a 40-hour workweek with overtime for any hours exceeding 40. Joe typically works 9 hours per day, Monday through Thursday, and 4 hours on Friday. He then flies home for the weekend. After several months, he discovers the hospital is billed for 44 to 48 hours per week almost every week. Joe confronts the company billing department because this practice conflicts with the tenet of the AHIMA Code of Ethics that states that health information management professionals:

    a. Respect the rights and dignity of all individuals

    b. Adhere to the vision, mission, and values of the association

    c. Promote and protect the confidentiality and security of health records and health information

    d. Refuse to participate in or conceal unethical practices or procedures

130. Agreements that are reached in a participant agreement or vendor contract should be developed into:

    a. Operational policies

    b. Strategy plans

    c. Admit, discharge, transfer notifications

    d. Long-term vision for technical interoperability

131. The process of reviewing and validating a physician's education and experience prior to granting medical staff membership is called:

    a. Outcomes management

    b. Credentialing

    c. Surveillance

    d. Utilization review

132. Which of the following would be an indicator of process problems in a health information department?

    a. 5% decline in the number of patients who indicate satisfaction with hospital care

    b. 10% increase in the average length of stay

    c. 15% reduction in bed turnover rate

    d. 18% error rate on abstracting data

133. Which of the following is a true statement about business process reengineering?

    a. It is intended to make small incremental changes to improve a process.

    b. It seeks to reevaluate and redesign organizational processes to make dramatic performance improvements.

    c. It implies making few changes to achieve significant improvements in cost, quality, service, and speed.

    d. Its main focus is to reduce services.

134. Strategic thinkers exhibit which of the following skills?

    a. Discomfort with uncertainty and risk

    b. The ability to gain a powerful core of healthcare entity supporters and customers

    c. Flexibility but lacking creativity

    d. An ability to implement the vision and plan and be uncomfortable with change

135. For Medicare patients, how often must the home health agency's assessment and care plan be updated?

    a. At least every 60 days or as often as the severity of the patient's condition requires

    b. Every 30 days

    c. As often as the severity of the patient's condition requires

    d. Every 60 days

136. A set of activities designed to familiarize new employees with their jobs, the healthcare entity, and work culture is called:

    a. Training

    b. Job analysis

    c. Orientation

    d. Job rotation

137. Sarah, a coding manager, realizes that one of her long-term employees is experiencing a decrease in her coding quality. Sarah has counseled the employee several times and she has documented the issues and placed them in the employee's file. Sarah has been advised by her manager that she needs to initiate a performance improvement plan for the employee. The next step that Sarah needs to do is:

    a. Document performance issues

    b. Meet with the employee to review the performance improvement plan

    c. Develop an action plan incorporating SMART goals that will assist employee in achieving performance goals

    d. Review the performance improvement plan with the HIM manager and human resources

138. Kelly's husband is being transferred to a new position in another state. Kelly has to resign her position as director of HIM at Memorial Hospital, a job she has enjoyed for five years. This is an example of what type of employee turnover?

    a. Functional

    b. Voluntary

    c. Involuntary

    d. Separation

139. The following information was abstracted from Community Hospital's balance sheet.

Total assets	$25,000,000
Current assets	$4,000,000
Total liabilities	$10,000,000
Current liabilities	$5,000,000

A vendor selling a large dollar amount of goods to this hospital on credit would:

a. Not be concerned because total assets exceed total liabilities

b. Not be concerned because the debt ratio is less than one half

c. Be somewhat concerned because the current ratio is less than one

d. Not analyze the balance sheet because the vendor would care more about the income statement

140. Community Hospital is evaluating the following three investments. Which one has the highest profitability index?

	Radiology Investment	Cardiology Investment	Pharmacy Investment
Present value of cash inflows	$2,000,000	$1,200,000	$40,000
Present value of cash outflows	$500,000	$300,000	$10,000

a. Radiology investment

b. Cardiology investment

c. Pharmacy investment

d. All three are equally profitable

141. The HIM manager is developing performance standards for the analysts. The manager will use these performance standards in order to:

a. Assign daily work

b. Communicate performance expectations

c. Describe the elements of a job

d. Prepare a job advertisement

142. What type of healthcare organization review is conducted at the request of the healthcare facility seeking accreditation?

a. Vocational review

b. Compulsory review

c. Complimentary review

d. Voluntary review

143. A SWOT analysis created by the director of the HIM department indicates that all of the coding staff are credentialed and up to date on their continuing education credits. In a SWOT analysis, this would be considered a:

    a. Strength

    b. Weakness

    c. Opportunity

    d. Threat

144. Aaron's workspace is filled with notes posted to the walls regarding coding rules. He has even created file folders for coding tips according to body system. Aaron is most likely what type of sensory learner?

    a. Auditory

    b. Kinesthetic

    c. Tactile

    d. Visual

145. An accrediting agency's published rules, which serve as the basis for comparative assessment during the review or survey process, are called:

    a. Accreditation controls

    b. Accreditation guides

    c. Accreditation policies

    d. Accreditation standards

146. Contracting for staffing to handle a complete function within the HIM department, such as the Cancer Registry function, would be considered what type of contracting arrangement?

    a. Full-service

    b. Part-time

    c. Project-based

    d. Temporary

147. Dr. Smith, an OB-GYN specialist, has just become a staff member at Medical Center Hospital, where she may offer care and treatment related to obstetrics and gynecology including performing deliveries and gynecological surgery. The process of defining what services she may perform is called:

    a. Outcomes management

    b. Care mapping

    c. Granting privileges

    d. Retrospective review

148. Every year, a director of health information services sponsors a series of presentations about the confidentiality of patient information. All facility employees are required to attend a session. This method of educational delivery is called:

    a. Career development

    b. In-service education

    c. On-the-job training

    d. Orientation

149. In the HIM department at Memorial Hospital, each newly hired coder spends an afternoon with a medical biller. The coder follows the biller around as they complete job tasks to get an idea of how coding and billing impact one another. This is an example of what type of on-the-job training?

    a. Job rotation

    b. Job shadowing

    c. Cross-training

    d. Coaching

150. Identify the true statement regarding training.

    a. A variety of methods should be used to accommodate different learning styles.

    b. Training should be limited to the information system only.

    c. Training should be performed a minimum of six months prior to implementation of the information system.

    d. In order to facilitate training, all employees should receive the exact same training regardless of their position.

PRACTICE EXAM 2

Domain 1   *Data and Information Governance*

1. Which of the following outcomes most likely results from a data entry error in the MPI?

    a. John Stevenson was sent home with a prescription to continue 0.625 Digoxin instead of the 0.0625 dosage that he was initially prescribed.

    b. John Stevenson was assigned to room 1203 instead of 1213.

    c. John Stevenson was diagnosed with indigestion instead of appendicitis.

    d. John Stevenson was entered into the system as a new patient and assigned a new medical record number instead of being matched to the John W. Stevenson already in the system and keeping his current medical record number.

2. Who owns the health records of patients treated in a healthcare facility?

    a. The patient

    b. The third-party payer

    c. The facility

    d. The patient's family

3. In figuring a drug dosage, it is unacceptable to round up to the nearest gram if the drug is to be dosed in milligrams. Which dimension of data quality is being applied in this situation?

    a. Accuracy

    b. Granularity

    c. Precision

    d. Currency

4. Using the staff turnover information in the following graph, determine the next action the quality committee at the hospital should take.

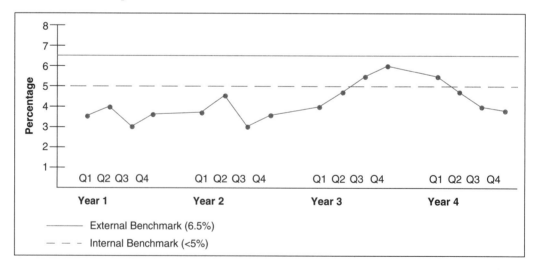

    a. Do nothing, as the data is below the external benchmark

    b. Coordinate a PI team to look into the cause for the high employee turnover rate in year 3

    c. Coordinate a PI team to look into the cause for the drop in employee turnover rate in year 4

    d. Do nothing, as the data is above the internal benchmark

5. The health information management (HIM) manager is concerned with a backlog in transcription of surgical reports. The medical staff rules and regulations stipulate that the surgeon should:

   a. Wait for the transcribed report

   b. Re-dictate the operative report

   c. Write a detailed postoperative progress note about the procedure performed

   d. Write a postoperative progress note that states the operative report has been dictated

6. One member of the medical staff reviewed a patient's history, examined the patient, and wrote findings and recommendations at the request of another member of the medical staff. The resulting medical report that documents the response of the reviewing medical staff member is a:

   a. Consultation report

   b. Discharge report

   c. History and physical exam

   d. Pathology report

7. The Abbreviated Injury Scale is a data element recorded in which of the following registries?

   a. Cancer

   b. Trauma

   c. Birth defects

   d. Immunization

8. Conducting an inventory of the facility's records, determining the format and location of record storage, assigning each record a time period for preservation, and destroying records that are no longer needed are all components of a:

   a. Case-mix index

   b. Master patient index

   c. Health record matrix

   d. Retention program

9. In establishing roles and responsibilities within a data governance program, which of the following would normally be embedded within an organization's business unit and be responsible for monitoring the data quality of the unit?

   a. Data content manager

   b. Data governance officer

   c. Data stakeholder

   d. Data steward

10. The director of the health information department wanted to determine the level of physicians' satisfaction with the department's services. The director surveyed the physicians who came to the department. What type of sample is this?

    a. Direct

    b. Positive

    c. Guided

    d. Convenience

11. Who is responsible for the content, quality, and authentication of the discharge summary?

    a. Attending physician

    b. Head nurse

    c. Consulting physician

    d. Admitting nurse

12. Under which circumstances may an updated entry be added to a patient's health record in place of a complete history and physical?

    a. When the patient is readmitted a second time for the same condition

    b. When the patient is readmitted within 30 days of the initial treatment for a different condition

    c. When the patient is readmitted a third time for the same condition

    d. When the patient is readmitted within 30 days of the initial treatment for the same condition

13. The HIM director wants to ensure that state regulations are being followed with regard to retention of the health records of minors. Which of the following data management domains would be responsible for ensuring these regulations are followed?

    a. Data architecture management

    b. Metadata management

    c. Data life cycle management

    d. Master data management

14. General Hospital is performing peer reviews of its medical providers for quality outcomes of care. The hospital has over 500 providers on its medical staff. The process to review even 10 cases for each provider is quite extensive. To accomplish this review process, it will review 20 percent of each provider's inpatient admissions to the hospital on an every-other-year rotation. Which of the following techniques has been applied to this review process?

    a. Benchmarking

    b. Data analysis

    c. Sampling

    d. Skewing

15. The clinical statement "microscopic sections of the gallbladder reveal a surface lined by tall columnar cells of uniform size and shape" would be documented on which health record form?

    a. Operative report

    b. Pathology report

    c. Discharge summary

    d. Nursing note

16. Standardizing medical terminology to avoid differences in naming various medical conditions and procedures (such as the synonyms bunionectomy, McBride procedure, and repair of hallux valgus) is one purpose of:

    a. Content and structure standards

    b. Security standards

    c. Transaction standards

    d. Vocabulary standards

17. As part of the initiative to improve data integrity, the Data Quality Committee conducted an inventory of all the hospital's databases. The review showed that more than 70 percent of the identified databases did not have data dictionaries. Given this data, what should be the committee's first action?

    a. Disregard the data

    b. Establish a data dictionary policy with associated standards

    c. Develop an in-service training program on data dictionary use

    d. Distribute a memorandum to all department heads on the value of a data dictionary

18. At Medical Center Hospital, the master patient index system is not meeting facility needs. There are duplicate numbers and errors in patient identification information. The IS director replaces the system with a newer system from a different vendor. After several months, the new system is exhibiting many of the same problems as the old system, and the facility staff is frustrated and angry. What is the most likely cause of the problem?

    a. The new system has the same design flaws as the previous system.

    b. The old system was not properly disabled and has infected the new system.

    c. Underlying human and process problems were not identified and corrected prior to making a system change.

    d. Human error is the cause of all of the problems with both systems.

19. Sue Smith has been admitted to Healthwise Hospital with stroke symptoms. Which professionals on her healthcare team are primarily responsible for documenting diagnosis and treatment information in her record during her hospital stay?

    a. Dr. Helms, her primary physician; and other providers on her care team

    b. Mrs. Hunter, the hospital CEO; and Dr. Henry, the medical director

    c. Mr. Charles, the HIM director

    d. Mr. Berry, the medical archive research director

20. A data element such as "date of birth" in a database is considered which of the following?

    a. Master data

    b. Metadata

    c. Structured data

    d. Unstructured data

21. The function that includes compiling the pertinent information from the health record, based on predetermined data sets, to enter into a separate database is called:

    a. Abstracting

    b. Data dictionary

    c. Data migration

    d. Analysis

22. A number assigned to patients in a cancer registry in the order that the patients are entered in the registry every year (for example, 03-0001) is a(n) _____ number.

    a. Accession

    b. Reference

    c. Follow-up

    d. Tracking

23. What information can be determined from the data in the following graph?

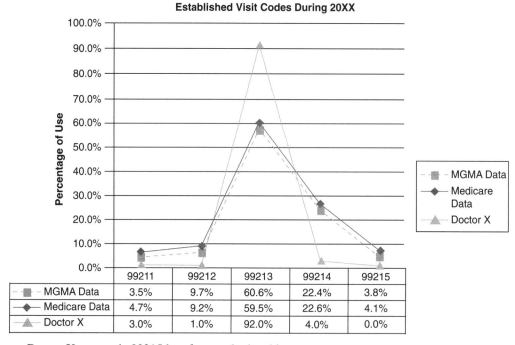

Established Visit Codes During 20XX

	99211	99212	99213	99214	99215
MGMA Data	3.5%	9.7%	60.6%	22.4%	3.8%
Medicare Data	4.7%	9.2%	59.5%	22.6%	4.1%
Doctor X	3.0%	1.0%	92.0%	4.0%	0.0%

    a. Doctor X uses code 99215 less frequently than his peers.

    b. Doctor X's documentation does not support the codes submitted.

    c. Doctor X overutilizes code 99213 as compared with the documentation.

    d. Doctor X overutilizes code 99212 as compared with his peers.

24. Mark Fielding, RHIA, is the new HIM director at St. Joseph's Hospital. Since it opened in 1960, this hospital has kept all health records in two rented warehouses that are located near the main hospital. The warehouse property is being sold, and the records will have to be moved to the hospital location. Before that happens, the CFO would like Mark to determine whether any of the records should be purged and destroyed. What is Mark's first step to determine if any records can be destroyed?

    a. Research all state and federal regulations related to record retention and develop a schedule

    b. Determine how much space is available to move the records into

    c. Purge all records that are more than 10 years old regardless of dates of service or patient age

    d. Destroy the records due to their age

25. Two clerks are abstracting data for a registry. When their work is checked, discrepancies are found between similar data abstracted by the two clerks. Which data quality component is lacking?

    a. Completeness

    b. Validity

    c. Reliability

    d. Timeliness

26. According to accreditation standards, which document must be placed in the patient's record before a surgical procedure may be performed?

    a. Admission record

    b. Physician's order

    c. Report of history and physical examination

    d. Discharge summary

27. The data in the following graph illustrate changes in a hospital's profile. What concerns might the hospital's quality council need to address based on these changes in their customer base?

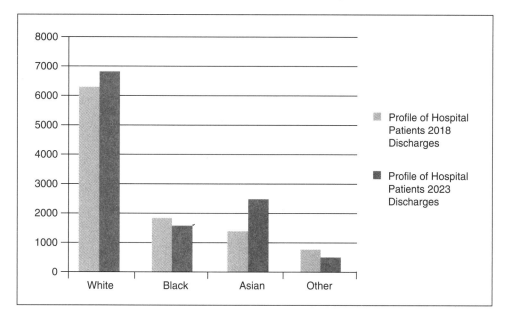

    a. Staffing changes might be necessary to accommodate patients who have cultural differences.

    b. Data collection has improved.

    c. No changes in staffing are necessary because the patient mix is appropriate.

    d. The quality council should ask for more detailed data.

Domain 2 *Compliance with Access, Use, and Disclosure of Health Information*

28. George is going to Arizona for the winter. What will offer him secure, online, 24-hour access to his personal health information from University Hospital System in the Midwest regardless of where he is, as long as he has an internet connection?

    a. Personal health record

    b. Telecommuting

    c. Patient portal

    d. Telehealth

29. How would you respond if a patient came to you with questions about how his or her health information is used?

    a. Show the patient the notice of privacy practices

    b. Refer the patient to his or her physician

    c. Show the patient the organization's mission and vision

    d. Refer the patient to the organization's marketing department

30. Which of the following individuals may authorize release of health information?

    a. An 86-year-old patient with a diagnosis of advanced dementia

    b. A married 15-year-old father

    c. A 15-year-old minor

    d. The parents of an 18-year-old student

31. At a recent medical staff committee meeting, a committee member asked what the state laws are for breach notification and how these laws will impact facility policy. The HIM director explained to the committee member that the state laws for breach notification are _____ and therefore may not guide facility policies related to breach notification for medical information.

    a. Generally tailored to medical information

    b. Generally not tailored to medical information

    c. Generally created in response to wrongful disclosures of medical information

    d. Generally nonexistent

32. Under what access security mechanism would an individual be allowed access to ePHI if he or she has a proper login and password, belongs to a specified group, and his or her workstation is located in a specific place within the facility?

    a. Role-based

    b. User-based

    c. Context-based

    d. Job-based

33. A physician office is implementing a vendor's personal health record system to be used by a majority of patients in order to help improve the office's achievement of value-based care. What technology would help facilitate this goal?

    a. Patient portal

    b. Preadmission system

    c. Clinical database

    d. Chart conversion

34. The process of entity authentication means a computer:

    a. Prevents rebooting to deactivate a log-off system

    b. Reads a predetermined set of criteria to determine if a user is who he or she claims to be

    c. Allows rebooting to activate a sign-in process

    d. Rejects multiple logins

35. The security devices situated between the routers of a private network and a public network to protect the private network from unauthorized users are called:

    a. Audit trails

    b. Passwords

    c. Firewalls

    d. Encryptors

36. The compliance officer received an automated alert that a user accessed the PHI of a patient with the same last name as the user. This is an example of a(n):

    a. Authentication

    b. Trigger

    c. Transmission security

    d. Integrity

37. What is the most common type of security threat to a health information system?

    a. External to the healthcare entity

    b. Internal to the healthcare entity

    c. Environmental in nature

    d. Computer viruses

38. On review of the audit log for an EHR system, the HIM director discovers that a departmental employee with authorized access to patient records is printing far more records than the average user. In this case, what should the supervisor do?

    a. Reprimand the employee

    b. Fire the employee

    c. Determine what information was printed and why

    d. Revoke the employee's access privileges

39. Under the HIPAA privacy standard, which of the following types of protected health information (PHI) must be specifically identified in an authorization?

    a. History and physical reports

    b. Operative reports

    c. Consultation reports

    d. Psychotherapy notes

40. Community Hospital is discussing restricting the access that physicians have to electronic clinical records. The medical record committee is divided on how to approach this issue. Some committee members maintain that all information should be available; whereas, others maintain that HIPAA restricts access. The HIM director is part of the committee. Which of the following statements should the director advise to the committee?

    a. HIPAA restricts physician access to all information.

    b. The "minimum necessary" concept does not apply to disclosures made for treatment purposes; therefore, physician access should not be restricted.

    c. The "minimum necessary" concept does not apply to disclosures made for treatment purposes, but the healthcare entity must define what physicians need as part of their treatment role.

    d. The "minimum necessary" concept applies only to attending physician; therefore, restriction of access must be implemented.

41. Per the HIPAA Privacy Rule, which of the following requires authorization for research purposes?

    a. Use of Mary's deidentified information about her myocardial infarction

    b. Use of Mary's information about her asthma in a limited data set

    c. Use of Mary's individually identifiable information related to her asthma treatments

    d. Use of medical information about Jim, Mary's deceased husband

42. What information process must the legal counsel of Smithville Hospital perform to prepare for a lawsuit against the hospital?

    a. Information governance

    b. E-Discovery

    c. Transparency

    d. Enterprise information management

43. City Hospital's HIPAA committee is considering a change in policy to allow hospital employees who are also hospital patients to access their own patient information in the hospital's EHR system. A committee member notes that HIPAA provides rights to patients to view their own health information. However, another member wonders if this action might present other problems. In this situation, what suggestion should the HIM director provide?

    a. HIPAA requires that employees have access to their own information, so privileges should be granted to the employees to perform this function.

    b. HIPAA does not allow employees to have access to their own information, so the policy should not be implemented.

    c. Allowing employees to access their own records using their job-based access rights appears to violate HIPAA's minimum necessary requirement; therefore, allow employees to access their records through normal procedures.

    d. Employees are considered a special class of people under HIPAA and the policy should be implemented.

44. Johnny is 12 years old and his parents are divorced. In order for Johnny to receive medical treatment, generally:

    a. Both parents must consent

    b. One parent must consent

    c. A court-appointed guardian must consent

    d. Johnny can consent

45. A plaintiff's attorney has requested "any and all records" of his client, a former patient at General Hospital. The hospital may interpret this request to:

    a. Include e-mail messages between the patient and General Hospital providers

    b. Include only information maintained on paper

    c. Exclude text messages between the patient and General Hospital providers

    d. Exclude calendar files

46. A patient requests that disclosures made from her medical record be limited to specific clinical notes and reports. Given HIPAA requirements, how must the hospital respond?

    a. The hospital must accept the request but does not have to agree to it.

    b. The hospital must honor the request.

    c. The hospital must guarantee that the request will be followed.

    d. The hospital must agree to the request, providing that state or federal law does not prohibit it.

47. An employee forgot his user ID badge at home and uses another employee's badge to access the computer system. What controls should have been in place to minimize this security breach?

    a. Access controls

    b. Security incident procedures

    c. Security management process

    d. Workforce security awareness training

48. The process of releasing health record documentation originally created by a different provider is called:

    a. Privileged communication

    b. Subpoena

    c. Jurisdiction

    d. Redisclosure

49. Today, Janet Kim had her first appointment with a new dentist. She was not presented with a Notice of Privacy Practices. Is this acceptable?

    a. No, a dentist is a healthcare clearinghouse, which is a covered entity under HIPAA.

    b. Yes, a dentist is not a covered entity per the HIPAA Privacy Rule.

    c. No, it is a violation of the HIPAA Privacy Rule.

    d. Yes, the Notice of Privacy Practices is not required.

50. Mercy Hospital personnel need to review the health records of Katie Grace for utilization review purposes (#1). They will also be sending her records to her physician for continuity of care (#2). Under HIPAA, these two functions are:

    a. Use (#1) and disclosure (#2)

    b. Request (#1) and disclosure (#2)

    c. Disclosure (#1) and use (#2)

    d. Disclosures (#1 and #2)

51. Jennifer's widowed mother is elderly and often confused. She has asked Jennifer to accompany her to physician office visits because she often forgets to tell the physician vital information. Under the Privacy Rule, the release of her mother's PHI to Jennifer is:

    a. Never allowed

    b. Allowed when the information is directly relevant to Jennifer's involvement in her mother's care or treatment

    c. Allowed only if Jennifer's mother is declared incompetent by a court of law

    d. Allowed access to PHI; any family member is always allowed access to PHI

Data Analytics and Informatics

52. What is the primary difference between a closed and an open system?

    a. Closed systems are designed for use in secure environments whereas the open system can operate in any environment

    b. Closed systems do not interact with the environment while open systems are influenced by the environment

    c. A closed system is for internal use only while the open system works with the Internet

    d. A closed system costs money whereas the open system is free

53. In the modern systems development life cycle (SDLC), performing change management is initiated in which of the following phases?

    a. Design or acquire

    b. Develop or implement

    c. Identification of need

    d. Monitor results

54. What relationships is the following entity relationship diagram showing?

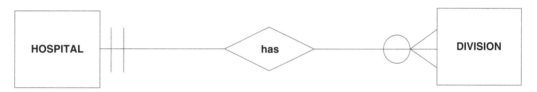

    a. Each division has one hospital, but each hospital has many divisions.

    b. Each hospital has one division, but each division has many hospitals.

    c. Each hospital has one division, and each division has one hospital.

    d. Each division has one hospital, and each hospital has one division.

55. The computer-based process of extracting, quantifying, and filtering data that reside in a database is called:

    a. Autocoding

    b. Bar coding

    c. Data mining

    d. Intelligent character recognition

56. Systems linked by _____ allow HIE participants to search for health records on each of the other systems using patient indexing and identification software.

    a. ADTs

    b. APIs

    c. CCDs

    d. RLSs

57. The distribution in this curve is:

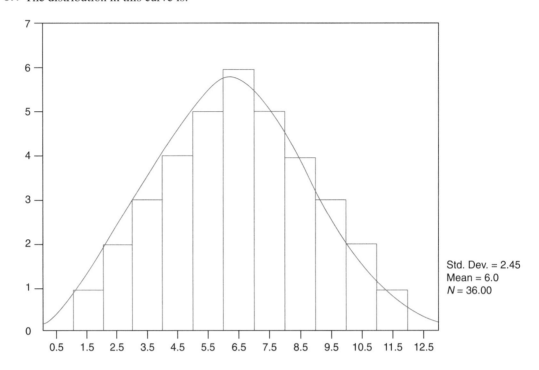

Std. Dev. = 2.45
Mean = 6.0
N = 36.00

   a. Skewed left

   b. Bimodal

   c. Normal

   d. Skewed right

58. Dr. Anderson orders 500 mg of penicillin by mouth three times a day for Jane Carlson, who is being seen in the hospital emergency department. The computer sends an alert to Dr. Anderson to tell her the patient, Jane Carlson, is allergic to penicillin. What type of computer system is Dr. Anderson using?

   a. Clinical data repository

   b. Data exchange standard

   c. Clinical decision support

   d. Health informatics standard

59. The nurse manager on the internal medicine unit of the hospital noticed that Dr. Winters in the ED admits many patients to the internal medicine unit. She is wondering if he admits patients to the hospital from the ED more often than other physicians. What type of analysis should be done to answer her question?

   a. Data warehousing

   b. Data governance

   c. Data mining

   d. Data modeling

60. When a healthcare professional complains that the EHR produces too many alerts, action should be taken to:

    a. Dismiss the complaint because data quality will be impacted without the alerts

    b. Eliminate some of the alerts about which most professionals have complained

    c. Retrain the professional on how to use alerts correctly and monitor for future issues

    d. Set up a process to evaluate and correct alert fatigue overall for the EHR

61. Using the admission criteria provided, determine if the following patient meets severity of illness and intensity of service criteria for admission.

Severity of Illness	Intensity of Service
Persistent fever	Inpatient-approved surgery or procedure within 24 hours of admission
Active bleeding	Intravenous medications or fluid replacement
Wound dehiscence	Vital signs every 2 hours or more often

    John Smith presents to the emergency room at 1500 hours with a fever of 101 degrees F, which he has had for the last three days. He was discharged six days ago following a colon resection. X-rays show a bowel obstruction and the plan is to admit him to surgery in the morning.

    a. The patient does not meet both severity of illness and intensity of service criteria.

    b. The patient does meet both severity of illness and intensity of service criteria.

    c. The patient meets intensity of service criteria but not severity of illness criteria.

    d. The patient meets severity of illness criteria but not intensity of service criteria.

62. This type of data display tool is a plotted chart of data that shows the progress of a process over time.

    a. Bar graph

    b. Histogram

    c. Pie chart

    d. Line graph or plot

63. As part of a large PI initiative that is occurring in a hospital, the PI team is tasked with presenting their findings to hospital administration. The PI team presents data on the number of urinary tract infections (UTIs) that were documented and coded at the facility. Hospital administration finds this information interesting but are unclear as to what the data means to the organization. Why is the hospital administration unclear about this data?

    a. Although the data provides important information regarding infections, the context of the data was missing from the presentation.

    b. Although the data seems important, administration is confused about why a PI team in concerned with UTIs.

    c. PI teams do not typically report their findings within the organization, so this presentation confused administration.

    d. PI teams are rarely concerned with clinical quality metrics and are only concerned with workflow issues.

64. In understanding the characteristics of information systems, what must be present to tie component objects together?

    a. Attributes

    b. Boundaries

    c. Relationships

    d. Unity of purpose

65. Which of the following is an operational element that should be included in a migration path for a hospital with an existing EHR and wishing to improve its population health data for value-based care reimbursement?

    a. Acquisition of a clinical data warehouse

    b. Building a data dictionary that encompasses data needs across the continuum

    c. Coordinating the collection and use of social determinants of health

    d. Supporting e-prescribing from computerized provider order entry systems

66. A hospital is undergoing a major reconstruction project and a new director of nursing has been hired. At the same time, the nursing documentation component of the EHR has been implemented. The fact that nursing staff satisfaction scores have risen is:

    a. A result of anecdotal benefits of EHR

    b. A result of qualitative benefits of EHR

    c. A result of reconfiguration of the nursing units

    d. Uncertain due to existence of confounding variables

67. Training "super" users who assist other end users in learning a new information system occurs in which step of the system development life cycle?

    a. Acquisition

    b. Implementation

    c. Maintenance

    d. Specification of requirements

68. There were 25 inpatient deaths, including newborns, at Community Memorial Hospital during the month of June. The hospital performed five autopsies during the same period. The gross autopsy rate for the hospital for June was:

    a. 0.02%

    b. 0.2%

    c. 5%

    d. 20%

69. Community Memorial Hospital discharged nine patients on April 1st. The length of stay for each patient is shown in the following table. What is the mode length of stay for this group of patients?

Patient	Number of Days
A	1
B	5
C	3
D	3
E	8
F	8
G	8
H	9
I	9

   a. 5 days

   b. 6 days

   c. 8 days

   d. 9 days

70. The HIM manager is reviewing third-quarter data from the previous year to identify patterns of patient admissions. The manager then uses this data to forecast expected patient admissions in order to determine coding and analyst staffing needs for this year. What technique is the HIM manager using?

   a. Descriptive statistics

   b. Inferential statistics

   c. Predictive modeling

   d. Data modeling

71. A doctor is reviewing lab results on a patient in his office. The EHR screen displays one set of results in red with a flashing asterisk and also shows that this result is three times higher than the expected value. This is an example of a(n):

   a. Alert

   b. Dashboard

   c. Structured data

   d. Unstructured data

72. Over the last 10 years, the number of ICU beds in your state decreased by 20 percent. How might this trend impact your tertiary-level healthcare facility?

   a. There would be no impact as the number of inpatient beds at your facility remains the same.

   b. The volume of patients in your ICU has the potential to increase.

   c. There would be no impact because inpatient stays are no longer reimbursed by Medicare.

   d. The volume of patients in your ICU has the potential to decrease.

73. What architectural model of health information exchange allows participants to access data in point-to-point exchange?

    a. Consolidated

    b. Federated—consistent databases

    c. Federated—inconsistent databases

    d. Switch

74. Which of the following basic services provided by an HIE entity ensures that information can be retrieved as needed?

    a. Consent management

    b. Person identification

    c. Registry and directory

    d. Secure data transport

75. Which of the following characteristics of information systems is most often overlooked in implementing health IT?

    a. Hardware and other equipment

    b. Principles on which people perform their work

    c. Relationships between software and hardware

    d. Software functionality

76. What term is used to describe the ability of one hospital's EHR from Vendor ABC to communicate flawlessly with another hospital's EHR from Vendor XYZ without any glitches or loss of data integrity?

    a. Interoperability

    b. Electronic health record

    c. Health information technology

    d. Health information exchange

77. A report developed by a PI team on the occurrence of methicillin-resistant *Staphylococcus aureus* infection in a neonatal intensive care unit was subsequently used by the perinatal morbidity and mortality committee in a monthly review of infant morbidity. Access to this report was possible because it was housed in the organization's:

    a. Information warehouse

    b. Comparative performance data

    c. PI database

    d. Computer hard drive

78. Healthright Clinic, a large IDS, is evaluating the processes of patient care and patient outcomes in pediatrics. It is using software to help solve problems and check if the care given meets established guidelines. What method or tool is in the software that helps in this process?

    a. Algorithms

    b. Data warehouses

    c. Data repositories

    d. Scheduling

79. Community Hospital uses barcoding technology as part of its medication management processes. Barcoding is an example of:

    a. Radio frequency identification technology

    b. Character and symbol recognition technology

    c. Voice recognition technology

    d. Vector graphic data

80. A major barrier to fully interoperable health information systems has been:

    a. Federal government mandate

    b. Lack of interoperability standards

    c. Meaningful use incentive program

    d. Proprietary nature of vendor products

81. Physicians use the _____ to access multiple sources of patient information within the healthcare organization's network.

    a. Data repository

    b. Clinical information system

    c. Data warehouse

    d. Clinician web portal

82. Which graph is the best choice to use when comparing lengths of stay across three hospitals?

    a. Line graph

    b. Bar graph

    c. Pie chart

    d. Scatter diagram

83. This analytic technique is being used by CMS to assist in prepayment audits.

    a. Descriptive statistics

    b. Graphical analysis

    c. Exploratory data analysis

    d. Predictive modeling

84. The relationship between patient gender and readmission to the hospital is best displayed using a:

    a. Frequency chart

    b. Contingency table

    c. Bar chart

    d. Pie chart

85. In which phase of the modern systems development life cycle does the disposal of out-of-date system components occur?

    a. Monitoring of results

    b. Identification of need

    c. Maintenance

    d. Implementation

Domain 4 *Revenue Cycle Management*

86. A coding audit shows that an inpatient coder is using multiple codes that describe the individual components of a procedure rather than using a single code that describes all the steps of the procedure performed. Which of the following should be done in this case?

    a. Require all coders to implement this practice

    b. Report the practice to the OIG

    c. Counsel the coder to stop the practice immediately

    d. Put the coder on an unpaid leave of absence

87. The patient accounting department at Wildcat Hospital is concerned because last night's bill drop contained half the usual number of inpatient cases. Which of the following reports will be most useful in determining the reason for the low volume of bills?

    a. Accounts receivable aging report

    b. Discharged, not final billed report

    c. Case-mix index report

    d. Discharge summary report

88. In order to determine the hospital's expected MS-DRG payment, the hospital's blended rate is multiplied by the MS-DRG's _____ to determine the dollar amount paid.

    a. Case-mix number

    b. Relative weight

    c. Major diagnostic category

    d. Length of stay

89. Assign codes for the following scenario: A 35-year-old male is admitted with esophageal reflux. An esophagoscopy and closed esophageal biopsy were performed.

> K20.90   Esophagitis, unspecified without bleeding
>
> K20.91   Esophagitis, unspecified with bleeding
>
> K21.00   Gastro-esophageal reflux disease with esophagitis, without bleeding
>
> K21.01   Gastro-esophageal reflux disease with esophagitis, with bleeding
>
> K21.9   Gastro-esophageal reflux disease without esophagitis

Section	Body System	Root Operation	Body Part	Approach	Device	Qualifier
Medical and Surgical	Gastrointestinal System	Inspection	Upper Intestinal Tract	Via Natural or Artificial Opening Endoscopic	No Device	No Qualifier
0	D	J	0	8	Z	Z

Section	Body System	Root Operation	Body Part	Approach	Device	Qualifier
Medical and Surgical	Gastrointestinal System	Excision	Esophagus	Via Natural or Artificial Opening Endoscopic	No Device	Diagnostic
0	D	B	5	8	Z	X

Section	Body System	Root Operation	Body Part	Approach	Device	Qualifier
Medical and Surgical	Gastrointestinal System	Excision	Esophagus	Via Natural or Artificial Opening Endoscopic	No Device	Diagnostic
0	D	B	5	8	Z	Z

a. K21.9, 0DB58ZX

b. K20.90, 0DB58ZZ

c. K21.00, 0DB58ZX

d. K21.9, 0DJ08ZZ, 0DB58ZX

90. Which data collection program is the basis for the CMS value-based purchasing program?

a. Leapfrog

b. HEDIS

c. Care Compare

d. HCUP

91. In the Hospital Value-Based Purchasing Program, a facility's total performance score (TPS) is used to determine the amount of holdback dollars the facility has earned. In regard to the TPS, which is better?

a. A higher TPS is better.

b. A lower TPS is better.

c. A consistent TPS is better.

d. A downward trend in TPS is better.

92. Which type of identity theft occurs when a patient uses another person's name and insurance information to receive healthcare benefits?

    a. Criminal

    b. Financial

    c. Health

    d. Medical

93. John Baker has group health insurance coverage through his employer. John's household includes his spouse, two natural children (ages 30 and 15), an adopted child (age 7), and John's mother (age 64). Who may be included under dependent coverage in the health insurance policy?

    a. Spouse; natural child, age 15; and adopted child, age 7

    b. Spouse and natural child, age 30

    c. Spouse; two natural children, ages 30 and 15; and adopted child, age 7, and his mother

    d. Everyone in the household

94. How do providers benefit from the health insurance exchanges created under the Affordable Care Act?

    a. Providers should see an increase in reimbursement both from newly insured patients and from patients who are now eligible for Medicaid under the expanded programs.

    b. The ACA is a revenue-neutral act and therefore has no impact on provider reimbursement.

    c. The exchanges are about insurance, not reimbursement, so providers are not affected.

    d. Providers may see an increase in reimbursement but only from cases that historically would have been charity care.

95. In developing a coding compliance program, which of the following would *not* be ordinarily included as participants in coding compliance education?

    a. Current coding personnel

    b. Medical staff

    c. Newly hired coding personnel

    d. Nursing staff

96. Aging of accounts is the practice of counting the days, generally in increments, from the time a bill has been sent to the payer to the current day. What is the standard increment, in days, that most healthcare entities use for the aging of accounts?

    a. 7-day increment

    b. 14-day increment

    c. 30-day increment

    d. 90-day increment

97. What is the benefit of comparing the coding assigned by coders to the coding that appears on the claim?

    a. May find that more codes are required to support the claim

    b. May find that the charge description master soft coding is inaccurate

    c. Serves as a way for HIM to take over the management of patient financial services

    d. May find claim generation issues that cannot be found in other ways

98. When documentation in the health record is not clear, the coding professional should:

    a. Query the physician who originated the progress note or other report in question

    b. Refer to dictation from other encounters with the patient to get clarification

    c. Submit the question to the coding clinic

    d. Query a physician who consistently responds to queries in a timely manner

99. Using the information provided, this participating physician, who accepts assignment, can expect how much reimbursement from Medicare?

Physician's normal charge = $340
Medicare fee schedule = $300
Patient has met his deductible

    a. $140

    b. $240

    c. $300

    d. $340

100. The patient is a 47-year-old. What is the correct code for an initial inguinal herniorrhaphy for incarcerated hernia?

    a. 49496, Repair, initial inguinal hernia, full-term infant younger than age 6 months, or preterm infant older than 50 weeks post conception age and younger than age 6 months at the time of surgery, with or without hydrocelectomy; incarcerated or strangulated

    b. 49501, Repair initial inguinal hernia, age 6 months to younger than 5 years, with or without hydrocelectomy; incarcerated or strangulated

    c. 49507, Repair initial inguinal hernia, age 5 years or older; incarcerated or strangulated

    d. 49521, Repair recurrent inguinal hernia, any age; incarcerated or strangulated

101. Following a motor vehicle accident, a patient presents to the emergency department (ED) with obvious head trauma and lower abdominal pain. The patient also notes recent hematuria prior to the accident and has a slight fever. A CT brain scan reveals the presence of a skull fracture with a hematoma, and the patient is admitted. During the hospital stay, the patient is treated for a urinary tract infection. The coder assigns the skull fracture and hematoma as present on admission, and the urinary tract infection as not present on admission. The coding manager reviews this case and identifies the following error:

    a. The urinary tract infection developed after admission, so it should not have been identified as present on admission.

    b. The urinary tract infection was not documented in the ED, so it cannot be identified as present on admission.

    c. No error was made, as the urinary tract infection was not present on admission.

    d. The urinary tract infection was present on admission because fever and hematuria were documented in the ED, so the coder was incorrect by not identifying it as present on admission.

102. Which of the following statements provide the most appropriate reflection about national and local coverage determinations (NCDs and LCDs)?

    a. They define the standard of care that must be used to treat the patient's condition.

    b. They define the specific diagnosis that supports medical necessity.

    c. They exist for all procedures and services that are provided to patients.

    d. They do not directly affect whether payment is received for the services provided.

103. The most recent coding audit has revealed a tendency to miss secondary diagnoses that would have increased the reimbursement for the case. Which of the following strategies will help to identify and correct these cases in the short term?

    a. Focus reviews on lower-weighted MS-DRGs from triples and pairs

    b. Identify the facility's top 10 to 15 APCs by volume and charges

    c. Contract with a larger consulting firm to do audits and education

    d. Focus reviews on surgical complications

104. Dr. Peters, a surgeon at Community Hospital, is trying to understand how she can help the hospital improve reimbursement from Medicare. The HIM manager explains to Dr. Peters that reducing catheter-associated UTIs and surgical site infections would improve the hospital's scores in which of the following domains of the Medicare Value-Based Purchasing program?

    a. Safety

    b. Clinical Care

    c. Efficiency and Cost Reduction

    d. Person/Community Engagement

105. When the physician does not specify the method used to remove a lesion during an endoscopy, what action should the coder take?

    a. Assign the removal by snare technique code

    b. Assign the removal by hot biopsy forceps code

    c. Assign the ablation code

    d. Query the physician as to the method used

106. Which of the following is a form of prospective reimbursement?

    a. Balance billing

    b. Fee-for service

    c. Per diem payment

    d. Capitation

107. Code the following scenario: A patient is admitted with major depression, recurrent, severe.

F32.9	Major depressive disorder, single episode, unspecified
F33.2	Major depressive disorder, recurrent, severe, without psychotic features
F33.3	Major depressive disorder, recurrent, severe, with psychotic symptoms
F33.9	Major depressive disorder, recurrent, unspecified

    a. F33.3

    b. F33.2

    c. F32.9

    d. F33.9

108. After a claim has been filed with Medicare, a healthcare entity had late charges posted to a patient's outpatient account that changed the calculation of the ambulatory payment classification (APC). What is the best practice for this entity to receive the correct reimbursement from Medicare?

    a. Nothing, because the claim has already been submitted

    b. Bill the patient for any remaining balance after payment from Medicare is received

    c. Submit an adjusted claim to Medicare

    d. Return the account to coding for review

109. At what point do most facilities begin counting days in accounts receivable?

    a. Date the patient registers

    b. Date the patient is discharged

    c. Date the claim drops

    d. Date the claim is received by the payer

110. Why are revenue audit functions necessary in organizations?

    a. To determine if reimbursement received is accurate based on the terms of the payer contract or agreement for all payment relationships

    b. To identify all individual claims in which an appeals process should be initiated

    c. To determine if claims are missing required data elements for submission

    d. To determine the best approach to focusing efforts on the largest denials

111. Which of the following is a goal for a clinical documentation integrity program?

    a. Allow coding directly from nursing notes

    b. Identifying missing, conflicting, or nonspecific documentation

    c. Identifying situations when a leading query is acceptable

    d. Allow billing for unbundled services

112. A polyp was removed from a patient's colon during an outpatient colonoscopy procedure. The physician and pathologist document the polyp as probable adenocarcinoma of the colon. The coder assigned the diagnosis code for adenocarcinoma of the colon. During an audit, the coding manager reviewed the coding assignment for this case and determined that the accurate coding assignment should have been which of the following?

    a. The coder should have assigned the diagnosis for the polyp.

    b. The coder should have assigned the diagnosis code for adenoma of the colon.

    c. The coder was correct in assigning the code for adenocarcinoma of the colon.

    d. The coding manager was unable to determine the correct code assignment and queried the physician.

113. A patient is admitted to the hospital with headache. After work-up the principal diagnosis is documented as cerebral hemorrhage. The patient also has anxiety, hypertension, and diabetes. In the inpatient prospective payment system, which of the following would determine the MDC assignment for this patient?

    a. Anxiety

    b. Cerebral hemorrhage

    c. Diabetes

    d. Hypertension

114. The facility's Medicare case-mix index has dropped, although other statistical measures appear constant. The CFO suspects coding errors. What type of coding audit review should be performed?

    a. Random audit

    b. Focused audit

    c. Compliance audit

    d. External audit

115. A comprehensive retrospective review should be conducted at least once a year of what aspect of the CDI program?

    a. Proficiency statistics

    b. Compliance issues

    c. All query opportunities

    d. Core key measures

116. When a payer rejects a claim for payment, organization staff must determine the reason for denial. If the denial was deemed due to eligibility determination, what process in the revenue cycle failed to operate as intended?

    a. Front-end process

    b. Middle process

    c. Back-end process

    d. Support services

117. Barbara is preparing a bill for a patient who has two different third-party payers. Verification of the payers has been performed. Before either of the payers can be billed, Barbara must:

    a. Determine which policy is primary and which is secondary

    b. Contact the attending physician

    c. Contact the patient

    d. Determine who is the primary policy holder

Management and Leadership

118. Maryann is implementing a new release of information (ROI) tracking system for her ROI clerks to utilize. She met with the vendor and the contract is pending until the legal department provides its final stamp of approval. Maryann is wondering what she should do next to introduce the process changes that need to take place and how she is going to manage the whole process. Maryann needs to develop a strong _____ plan in order for this process to be accepted by the HIM staff and for the entire project to be adopted smoothly.

    a. Negotiation

    b. Collaboration

    c. Conflict management

    d. Change management

119. CMS and the Joint Commission both require that healthcare professionals assess the work of colleagues in the same profession; this process is known as:

    a. Peer review

    b. Utilization review

    c. Workflow process

    d. Mediation

120. The process of conducting a thorough review of the internal and external conditions in which a healthcare entity operates is called:

    a. Environmental assessment

    b. Operations improvement planning

    c. Strategic management

    d. Employment assessment

121. The incidence of postoperative wound infections occurring in ORIF procedures in which antibiotics were and were not utilized is an example of which type of performance measure?

    a. Data measure

    b. Process measure

    c. Outcome measure

    d. System measure

122. What term is used to represent a difference between the budgeted amount and the actual amount of a line item that is not expected to reverse itself during a subsequent period?

    a. Permanent variance

    b. Fixed cost

    c. Temporary variance

    d. Flexible cost

123. Successful strategic managers understand that three competencies are common to all successful change and that these competencies can and must be developed. These three competencies are:

    a. Leadership, change management, and strategic development

    b. Organizational learning, visioning, and leadership

    c. Visioning, managing, and change management

    d. Improvement, visioning, and managing

124. A legally binding contract that draws from federal and local laws to define the requirements for participation in the eHealthExchange national network is:

    a. DIRECT exchange

    b. Blue Button

    c. Data Use and Reciprocal Support Agreement (DURSA)

    d. Trust Community

125. In order to expedite basic performance improvement team functioning, the team should:

    a. Use unstructured brainstorming

    b. Perform force field analysis

    c. Establish ground rules

    d. Use structured brainstorming

126. Identifying future health information needs for a healthcare entity and projecting specific initiatives required to meet those needs is part of:

    a. Data modeling

    b. Policy development

    c. Strategic planning

    d. Workflow modeling

127. Which discipline defines the natural laws of work and focuses on employee comfort and safety?

    a. Aesthetics

    b. Cybernetics

    c. Affinity grouping

    d. Ergonomics

128. Community Hospital is reviewing its job descriptions and notices that some job descriptions for clinical positions include a reference to the potential risks of exposure to blood-borne pathogens while others do not. The human resource manager insists that all job descriptions should include this language. Why is this important to include?

    a. It is not important, and the human resource manager is overstepping his or her role.

    b. Community Hospital needs to update job descriptions to meet HIPAA requirements.

    c. Community Hospital needs to define the level of risk for infection from blood-borne pathogens for its employees.

    d. Facilities are required to report incidences of HIV.

129. What type of organization works under contract with CMS to conduct Medicare and Medicaid certification surveys for hospitals?

    a. Accreditation organizations

    b. Certification organizations

    c. State licensure agencies

    d. Conditions of Participation agencies

130. Which of the following is a conflict management method in which both parties meet with an objective third party to explore their perceptions and feelings?

    a. Compromise

    b. Collaborative confrontation

    c. Control

    d. Constructive confrontation

131. The Hay method is used to measure the three levels of major compensable factors: the know-how, problem-solving, and accountability requirements of each position. This system is used for:

    a. Job evaluation

    b. Interviewing applicants

    c. Performance measurement

    d. Work scheduling

132. For a contract to be valid, it must include three elements. Which of the following is one of those elements?

    a. Assumption of risk

    b. Consideration

    c. Statute of limitations

    d. Notice of liability

133. One member of the coding staff requested to wear scrubs to work rather than street clothes, and this was approved by the section supervisor. Within a week, all members of the coding staff are now wearing scrubs to work. This is an example of _____:

    a. Stereotyping

    b. Affinity-attraction

    c. Affinity groups

    d. Bandwagon effect

134. A SWOT analysis created by the director of the HIM department indicates there is a local community college with an HIM program that could be a source of new coders for future open positions. In a SWOT analysis, this would be a(n):

    a. Strength

    b. Weakness

    c. Opportunity

    d. Threat

135. During a recent Joint Commission survey, one of the survey team members asked a nurse in the ICU about the medications that a patient was on and also asked for the nurse to explain how those medications were ordered and received from the pharmacy. After the nurse explained this process, the surveyor then went to the pharmacy and asked the pharmacist to explain his role in the medication process for this specific patient. The surveyor is utilizing which of the following processes?

a. Medication reconciliation

b. Document review

c. Drug diversion

d. Tracer methodology

Use the following information to answer questions 136 and 137.

Triad Healthcare Financial Data 12/31/201X	
Cash	$500,000
A/R	$250,000
Building	$1,000,000
Land	$700,000
A/P	$350,000
Mortgage	$600,000
Revenue	$2,500,000
Expenses	$2,250,000

136. Based on the financial data listed above, what was Triad's net income?

a. $150,000

b. $250,000

c. $400,000

d. $1,500,000

137. Based on the financial data listed, what was Triad's total net assets before posting net income for the year?

a. $250,000

b. $400,000

c. $1,250,000

d. $1,500,000

138. Caroline is interviewing candidates for a supervisor of release of information position. She asks each candidate to explain how they would prepare a record in answer to a subpoena. This is what type of interview question?

a. Behavior

b. Job knowledge

c. Situational

d. Work requirement

139. The HIM director hired an HIM data integrity analyst. This is a new position with a newly created job description. The director needs to develop performance standards for this job and will review a random selection of the job tasks performed in order to develop baseline data for future job performance assessments. This method is called:

    a. Benchmarking

    b. Work sampling

    c. Task interdependence

    d. Job complexity

140. The Health Information Services department at Medical Center Hospital has identified problems with its work processes. Too much time is spent on unimportant tasks, there is duplication of effort, and task assignment is uneven in quality and volume among employees. The manager has each employee complete a form identifying the amount of time he or she spends each day on various tasks. What is this tool called?

    a. Serial work distribution tool

    b. Work distribution chart

    c. Check sheet

    d. Flow process chart

141. Susan wants to become a privacy officer and is studying the examination workbook to prepare herself to take the test. She spends time in the evenings and on weekends, and she completes each chapter at her own pace. She feels she should be ready for the exam in six months. What type of learning model is Susan using?

    a. Blended

    b. Classroom

    c. Distance

    d. Self-directed

142. A distance learning method in which groups of employees in multiple classroom locations may listen to and see the material presented at the same time via satellite or telephone is called:

    a. Audio conferencing

    b. Computer-based training

    c. Videoconferencing

    d. Online learning

143. Which of the following is the process of meeting a prescribed set of standards or regulations to maintain active accreditation, licensure, or certification status?

    a. Compliance

    b. Deemed status

    c. Document review

    d. Performance improvement

144. How are employee performance standards used?

    a. To communicate performance expectations

    b. To assign daily work

    c. To describe the elements of a job

    d. To prepare a job advertisement

145. The use of simulation as a training technique is best suited for which of the following scenarios?

    a. Diversity training in an integrated health system covering a six-state area

    b. Disaster preparedness exercises

    c. Providing annual coding updates to physician office staff

    d. New employee orientation

146. Community Hospital is preparing to select an outsource company as a vendor for its release of information service. What is the first step that the hospital should initiate to gather information from each vendor under consideration?

    a. Engage in an RFP process

    b. Contact their legal department to review the contract

    c. Form a team to determine if a vendor is needed

    d. Facilitate a meet and greet with the administration and each potential vendor

147. Which of the following is a disadvantage of using off-site seminars or workshops as a learning model?

    a. On-site learning is generally more expensive than attending a seminar.

    b. Seminars are customized to each attendee's style of learning.

    c. Seminars are more expensive than on-site instruction.

    d. Seminars are usually poorly planned and organized.

148. Which process requires the verification of the educational qualifications, licensure status, and other experience of healthcare professionals who have applied for the privilege of practicing within a healthcare facility?

    a. Deemed status

    b. Judicial decision

    c. Subpoena

    d. Credentialing

149. The people or groups of people in an organization who will be affected by the project outcomes are the project's _____.

    a. Sponsors

    b. Stakeholders

    c. Staff

    d. Resources

150. Karen has two coders out on maternity leave, which has resulted in a coding backlog. She is working on a contract to reduce the coding backlog in order to maintain the organization's performance metrics for DNFB. This contract will allow her to hire staff until the coders return to work. What type of contract is Karen creating?

    a. Temporary

    b. Full service

    c. Emergency

    d. Long term

ANSWER KEY

Practice Question Answers

Domain 1 *Data and Information Governance*

1. **c** As data analysis tools have become more mature and the granularity of the data available in a healthcare entity increases, real-time analytics and performance improvement dashboards based on key performance indicators (KPIs) are becoming the norm. This analysis technique is used in this scenario by the coding manager (White 2020b, 523).

2. **c** Spoliation is a legal concept applicable to both paper and electronic records. When evidence is destroyed that relates to a current or pending civil or criminal proceeding, it is reasonable to infer that the party had a guilty conscience or another motive to avoid the evidence (Klaver 2017a, 87–88).

3. **a** A template-based data entry is a cross between structured and unstructured data entry. The user can pick and choose data that are entered frequently, thus requiring the entry of data that change from patient to patient. It assists the healthcare provider by providing directions in what needs to be documented One benefit of using a template is to ensure data integrity upon data entry (Sayles and Kavanaugh-Burke 2021, 19, 27).

4. **c** The Joint Commission requires that history and physicals be on patient charts within 24 hours of admission or before a surgical procedure. The turnaround time for the transcription service is problematic as the documentation is not in the record within the timeframe regulated by the Joint Commission (Reynolds and Morey 2020, 124).

5. **c** Correlation is a statistic that is used to describe the association or relationship between two variables (White 2020b, 516).

6. **a** Qualitative analysis is conducted to determine whether documentation is complete and includes all components set forth by CMS, state guidelines, and accrediting organization standards. Quantitative analysis determines whether required documentation is present in the chart or not (Reynolds and Morey 2020, 125–126).

7. **a** The federal government mandated the use of the Minimum Data Set (MDS) for Long-Term Care to plan the care of long-term care residents. The MDS 3.0 version became effective in 2010. This data set structures the assessment of long-term care residents in the following areas: delirium, cognitive loss and dementia, communication, vision function, activities of daily living function and rehabilitation potential, mood and behavior symptoms, activity-pursuit patterns, treatments and procedures, pain, and medications to name a few (Shaw and Carter 2019, 167).

8. **c** The claims data is secondary data, that is, the data are used for a purpose that was not the primary reason for collection (White 2020b, 520).

9. **d** Benchmarking is the systematic comparison of the products, services, and outcomes of one organization with those of a similar organization. Benchmarking comparisons also can be made using regional and national standards if the data collection processes are similar (Shaw and Carter 2019, 42).

10. **a** Concurrent record reviews help to catch incomplete documentation or unsigned orders while the patient is still in-house (Reynolds and Morey 2020, 125).

11. **d** Master patient indexes (MPI) contain important patient health information enabling facilities to retrieve patient health data quickly. The MPI allows a hospital to determine whether a patient has been seen in the facility before (Sharp and Madlock-Brown 2020, 177).

12. **b** Quantitative analysis is conducted to determine whether documentation is complete and accounted for in the medical record. If information is missing or incomplete, it is flagged for the provider to review and complete (Reynolds and Morey 2020, 125).

13. **d** The destruction of patient-identifiable clinical documentation should be carried out in accordance with relevant federal and state regulations and organizational policy. Electronic data can be destroyed with magnetic degaussing (demagnetizing) as this is an acceptable form of destruction for that medium. Burning, shredding, and pulverizing are acceptable destruction methods for paper-based records (Fahrenholz 2017b, 107).

14. **c** Duplicate health record numbers are when there is more than one unique identifier (for example, medical record number or person identifier) for the same person in the MPI. This causes one patient to have two or more different medical record numbers with the multihospital system, which would be an overlap (Reynolds and Morey 2020, 132–133).

15. **d** A dashboard report gives administration-structured information to make intelligent decisions for the future (Sayles and Kavanaugh-Burke 2021, 9).

16. **a** Only healthcare providers should document within the patient's record. However, HIM professionals can monitor documentation guidelines, train healthcare providers in documentation techniques and audit patient records (Reynolds and Morey 2020, 102).

17. **d** Financial data includes details about the patient's occupation, employer, and insurance coverage and is collected at the time of treatment. Healthcare providers use this data to complete claims forms that will be submitted to third-party payers (Fahrenholz 2017b, 74–76).

18. **c** Clinical laboratory reports should be reviewed to determine if a partial thromboplastin time (PTT) test was performed. Medication Administration Records (MAR) should be reviewed to determine if heparin was given after the PTT test was performed (Reynolds and Morey 2020, 114).

19. **c** In this example, DNFB met the benchmark in January, February, and June, which is 3/6 or 50 percent of the time (Handlon 2020, 253).

20. **a** The alternative hypothesis would complement the null. Here, it appears the null claims wait time is longer on weekends. Therefore, the alternative hypothesis would be (a). The wait time is shorter on weekends (White 2020b, 503).

21. **b** The data contained in the data dictionary are known as metadata. Metadata are descriptive data that characterize other data to create a clearer understanding of their meaning and to achieve greater reliability and quality of information (Sayles and Kavanaugh-Burke 2021, 21).

22. **b** Source systems are information systems that capture and feed data into the EHR. Source systems include the electronic medication administration record (EMAR), laboratory information system, radiology information system, hospital information system, nursing information systems, and more (Sayles and Kavanaugh-Burke 2021, 199).

23. **d**   Biomedical research is considered an ancillary function of the health record (Fahrenholz 2017b, 81–82).

24. **d**   The Uniform Ambulatory Care Data Set (UACDS) includes data elements specific to ambulatory care such as the reason for the encounter with the healthcare provider (Johns 2015, 280).

25. **b**   Medicare requires that all inpatient hospitals collect a minimum set of patient-specific data elements, which are in databases formulated from hospital discharge abstract systems. The patient-specific data elements are referred to as the Uniform Hospital Discharge Data Set (UHDDS) (Schraffenberger and Palkie 2022, 91–92).

26. **c**   Unstructured data is the use of free text or narrative data in the health record. It enables providers to document details and nuance that are usually not available with structured data. The main drawback to unstructured data entry centers on the general inability to determine the completeness of the data (Biedermann and Dolezel 2017, 159).

27. **b**   Care plans require documentation in a long-term care hospital (LTCH). Some LTCHs may use critical paths (or digipathways) for specific patients (James 2017a, 311).

28. **b**   Because of the risks associated with miscommunication, verbal orders are discouraged. When a verbal order is necessary, a clinician should sign, give his or her credentials (for example, RN, PT, or LPN), and record the date and time the order was received. Verbal orders for medication are usually required to be given to, and to be accepted only by, nursing or pharmacy personnel (Rinehart-Thompson 2017b, 178).

29. **b**   Examples of metadata include name of element, definition, application in which the data element is found, locator key, ownership, entity relationships, date first entered system, date terminated from system, and system of origin (Amatayakul 2017, 314–315).

30. **d**   Scatter diagrams are used to plot the points for two continuous variables that may be related to each other in some way. Whenever a scatter diagram indicates that the points are moving together in one direction or another, conclusions about the variables' relationship, either positive or negative, become evident. In this case a positive relationship between the variables can be seen as the points gather at the top of the diagram (Oachs 2020, 789).

31. **b**   The data flow for a hospital inpatient can begin in several ways. Data collection starts in the registration department if patients are a direct admission for their physician's office or hospital outpatient department. Data collection begins in the emergency room if the patients arrive at the hospital, are assessed in the emergency room, and are admitted as an inpatient. No matter where the data collection begins, the same patient demographic information is collected. During the course of the inpatient stay, patient care is delivered, and data is captured. As care is delivered and procedures are performed, charges are entered either by nursing staff or the personnel performing the procedure. After the patient is discharged, diagnosis and procedure codes are assigned (White 2021, 29-30).

32. **b**   Quantitative analysis is a review of the health record to identify deficiencies to ensure completeness and accuracy. It is generally conducted retrospectively, that is, after the patient's discharge from the facility or at the conclusion of treatment (Reynolds and Morey 2020, 125).

33. **b**   Every long-term care facility must complete a comprehensive assessment of every resident's needs by using the resident assessment instrument (RAI) (James 2017b, 325).

34. **d** A duplicate medical record number results in the creation of a new medical record for the patient. This duplicate number and the associated records results in a patient having medical information in disparate medical records that could impede proper care. Proper management of the MPI is critical to reduce or eliminate the assignment of duplicate medical record numbers (Reynolds and Morey 2020, 132-133).

35. **a** There are many types of patient-identifiable data elements that are pulled from the patient's healthcare record that are not included in the legal health record or designated record set definitions. Administrative data and derived data and documents are two examples of patient-identifiable data that are used in the healthcare organization. Administrative data are patient-identifiable data used for administrative, regulatory, healthcare operation, and payment (financial) purposes (Fahrenholz 2017a, 56).

36. **a** For the purposes of mapping, the term "coding system" is used very broadly to include classification, terminology, and other data representation systems. Mapping is necessary as health information systems and their use evolves in order to link disparate systems and data sets. Any data map will include a source and a target. The source is the code or data set from which the map originates (Biedermann and Dolezel 2017, 155).

37. **a** The digital signature is similar to the electronic signature except that it uses encryption to prove the authenticator's identity, which makes it most secure (Sayles and Kavanaugh-Burke 2021, 29).

38. **b** When entries are made in the health record regarding a patient who is particularly hostile or irritable, general documentation principles apply, such as charting objective facts and avoiding the use of personal opinions, particularly those that are critical of the patient. The degree to which these general principles apply is heightened because a disagreeable patient may cause a provider to use more expressive and inappropriate language. Further, a hostile patient may be more likely to file legal action in the future if the hostility is a personal attribute and not simply a manifestation of his or her medical condition (Rinehart-Thompson 2017b, 179).

39. **c** The provider is responsible for ensuring the quality of the documentation of the healthcare record (Rinehart-Thompson 2017b, 177).

40. **b** The HIM professional should advise the medical group practice to develop a list of statutes, regulations, rules, and guidelines regarding the release of the health record as the first step in determining the components of the legal health records (Rinehart-Thompson 2017b, 171–172).

41. **c** According to the UHDDS definition, ethnicity should be recorded on a patient record as Hispanic or Non-Hispanic. The UHDDS has been revised several times since 1986 (Schraffenberger and Palkie 2022, 91–92).

42. **b** The content of the resident assessment instruments (RAIs) is used to collect the necessary information from and about the facility resident. The RAI consists of three basic components: The Minimum Data Set (MDS), the Care Area Assessment (CAA) process, and the RAI utilization guidelines (James 2017b, 325).

43. **a** Authorship is the origination or creation of recorded information attributed to a specific individual or entity acting at a particular time. In other words, documentation in the EHR or other health record must be credited to the individual who created it. This is typically done through the use of a unique user identifier and a password (Sayles and Kavanaugh-Burke 2021, 29).

44. **c** The Uniform Ambulatory Care Data Set (UACDS) is a data set developed by NCVHS consisting of a minimum set of patient-specific or client-specific elements to be collected in ambulatory care settings. The purpose of the UACDS is to collect and report standardized ambulatory data (Johns 2015, 280).

45. **d** The quality of coded clinical data depends on a number of factors, including accuracy. Accuracy is ensuring that the coded data is free from error and a correct representation of the patient's diagnosis and procedures (Sharp and Madlock-Brown 2020, 202).

46. **b** The purpose of the data dictionary is to standardize definitions and ensure consistency of use. Standardizing data enhances use across systems. Communication is improved in clinical treatment, research, and business processes through a common understanding of terms (Sayles and Kavanaugh-Burke 2021, 41).

47. **c** An author is a person or system who originates or creates information that becomes part of the record. Each author must be granted permission by the healthcare entity to make such entries. Not all users will be granted authorship rights into all areas of the electronic health record (EHR). The individual must have the credentials required by state and federal laws to be granted the right to document observations and facts related to the provision of healthcare services. Authentication is a process by which a user (a person or entity) who authored an EHR entry or document is seeking to validate that they are responsible for the data contained within it (Biedermann and Dolezel 2017, 442–443).

48. **b** When erroneous entries are made in health records, policies and procedures should have provisions for how corrections are made. Educating clinicians who are authorized to document in the health record on the appropriate way to make corrections will promote consistency and standardization and maintain the integrity of the health record (Jenkins 2017, 161).

49. **b** An edit check is a standard feature in many applications' data entry and data collection software packages. Edit checks are preprogrammed definitions of each data field set up within the application. So, as data are entered, if any data are different from what has been preprogrammed, an edit message appears on the screen (Sayles and Kavanaugh-Burke 2021, 21).

50. **b** Providers must have a process in place for handling amendments, corrections, and deletions in health record documentation. An amendment is an alteration of the health information by modification, correction, addition, or deletion (Biedermann and Dolezel 2017, 448).

51. **c** Identity matching (also known as patient matching) is the process in which the facility identifies the right person within the database to exchange information between healthcare organizations. The process examines different demographic elements from different health information technology systems to determine if they refer to the same patient (Sayles and Kavanaugh-Burke 2021, 269).

52. **d** Authentication is the process of identifying the source of health record entries by attaching a handwritten signature, the author's initials, or an electronic signature and also the proof of authorship that ensures, as much as possible, that log-ins and messages from a user originate from an authorized source (Jenkins 2017, 159).

53. **a** Disaster recovery planning is the technological aspect of business continuity planning. HIM professionals assist in designing disaster recovery plans that address documenting information in the health record during down time or a disaster (Brinda and Watters 2020, 336).

54. c   The legal health record must meet accepted standards as defined by applicable federal regulations, state laws, and standards of accreditation agencies as well as the policies of the healthcare provider (Rinehart-Thompson 2017c, 171–172).

55. d   An advance directive is a written document that describes the patient's healthcare preferences in the event that he or she is unable to communicate directly at some point in the future. The types of advance directives vary by state but typically include living wills, healthcare surrogate designation, durable power of attorney for healthcare, and anatomical donation (James 2017a, 310).

56. b   Delinquent health records are those records that are not completed within the specified time frame, for example, within 14 days of discharge. A delinquent record is similar to an overdue library book. The definition of a delinquent chart varies according to the facility, but most facilities require that records be completed within 30 days of discharge as mandated by CMS regulations and Joint Commission standards. Some facilities require a shorter time frame for completing records because of concerns about timely billing (Reynolds and Morey 2020, 128).

57. a   Birth defects registries collect data on newborns with birth defects. Often population based, these registries serve a variety of purposes. For example, they provide information on the incidence of birth defects to study causes and prevention of birth defects, to monitor trends in birth defects to improve medical care for children with birth defects, and to target interventions for preventable birth defects such as folic acid to prevent neural tube defects (Sharp and Madlock-Brown 2020, 183).

58. c   Templates often provide clinical information by default and design. When used inappropriately, they may misrepresent a patient's condition and might not reflect changes in a condition. Unless the physician or other authorized provider removes the default documentation from the visit note, a higher level of service than is actually provided could be assigned (Jenkins 2017, 160–161).

59. c   Hybrid health records are increasingly seen as the most common transition points between fully paper and completely electronic records. Hybrid records may be a mixture of paper and electronic or multiple electronic systems that do not communicate or are not logically architected for record management (Biedermann and Dolezel 2017, 429).

60. b   An HIM professional must be aware of the retention statutes and retention periods in his or her state of employment and any federal statutes that apply. In some cases, the organization may define a retention period that is longer than the period required by the state. The organization should base its retention policy on hospital and medical needs and any applicable statutes and regulations (Reynolds and Morey 2020, 139).

61. a   The master patient index (MPI) is a permanent database including every patient ever admitted to or treated by the facility. Even though patient health records may be destroyed after legal retention periods have been met, the information contained in the MPI must be kept permanently (Reynolds and Morey 2020, 132).

62. d   In a trauma registry, the case definition might be all patients admitted with a diagnosis falling into ICD-10-CM code numbers S00–T88, the trauma diagnosis codes (Sharp and Madlock-Brown 2020, 181).

63. **d** The master patient index (MPI) is a permanent database including every patient ever admitted to or treated by the facility. Even though patient health records may be destroyed after legal retention periods have been met, the information contained in the MPI must be kept permanently (Reynolds and Morey 2020, 132).

64. **c** The health record is considered a primary data source because it contains patient-specific data and information about a patient that has been documented by the professionals who provided care or services to that patient (Fahrenholz 2017c, 128).

65. **c** Information governance is defined as ensuring leadership and organizational practices, resources, and controls for effective, compliant, and ethical stewardship of information assets to enable best clinical and business practices and serve patients, stakeholders, and the public good (Johns 2020, 75–77).

66. **a** In 1974, the federal government adopted the Uniform Hospital Discharge Data Set (UHDDS) as the standard for collecting data for the Medicare and Medicaid programs. When the Prospective Payment Act was enacted in 1983, UHDDS definitions were incorporated into the rules and regulations for implementing diagnosis-related groups (DRGs). A key component was the incorporation of the definitions of principal diagnosis, principal procedure, and other significant procedures, into the DRG algorithms (Amatayakul 2017, 301).

67. **d** Version control in healthcare is the process whereby a healthcare facility ensures that only the most current version of a patient's health record is available for viewing, updating, and so forth. However, there must be a way for authorized users to be able to view the previous version to see what was changed (Sayles and Kavanaugh-Burke 2021, 28).

68. **c** The Minimum Data Set for Long-Term Care is a federally mandated standard assessment form used to collect demographic and clinical data on nursing home residents. It consists of a core set of screening and assessment elements based on common definitions. To meet federal requirements, long-term care facilities must complete an MDS for every resident at the time of admission and at designated reassessment points throughout the resident's stay (James 2017b, 325–326).

69. **a** Common characteristics of data quality are relevancy, granularity, timeliness, currency, accuracy, precision, and consistency (Sharp and Madlock-Brown 2020, 202).

70. **a** Federal and state statutes, licensing requirements, and accreditation standards provide minimum guidelines to ensure accurate and complete documentation. Such documentation facilitates effective communication among caregivers to provide continuity of patient care, which is its primary purpose (Fahrenholz 2017e, 1).

71. **b** Planning for the eventual obsolescence of a technology is often not given high enough priority. Hardware obsolescence is a retention concern with electronic health records (EHRs). Record managers need to understand how long data will need to be migrated to ensure compliance with the long retention periods (years to decades) required for EHR systems (Biedermann and Dolezel 2017, 444)

72. **d** The integrity of each piece of data, including any document, must be ensured to maintain highly defensible business records. Document and data nonrepudiation are the methods by which the data are maintained in an accurate form after their creation, free of unauthorized changes, modifications, updates, or similar changes (Biedermann and Dolezel 2017, 443).

73. **a** The physician index categorizes patients by primary physician. It guides the retrieval of cases treated by a particular physician. This index is created simply by sorting patients by physician (Fahrenholz 2017c, 124).

74. **b** Case finding includes the methods used to identify the patients who have been seen and treated in the facility for the particular disease or condition of interest to the registry. After cases have been identified, extensive information is abstracted from the health record and entered into the registry database (Sharp and Madlock-Brown 2020, 179).

75. **c** When obtaining consent for treatment, the physician is the healthcare provider who would discuss the treatment with the patient. The basic elements of an informed consent should include the purpose of the proposed procedure, any risks associated with the procedure, and if any noninvasive treatment alternatives are available (Klaver 2017c, 141).

76. **d** A data dictionary is a descriptive list of the data elements to be collected in an information system or database whose purpose is to ensure consistency of terminology (Sharp and Madlock-Brown 2020, 203).

77. **d** Each facility must have a policy in place for dealing with situations where records remain incomplete for an extended period. The HIM director can be given authority to declare that a record is completed for purposes of filing when a provider relocates, dies, or has an extended illness that would prevent the record from ever being completed. Every effort should be made to have a partner or physician in the same specialty area complete the charts so that coding, billing, and statistical information are available (Reynolds and Morey 2020, 106).

78. **a** The stakeholder team will drive the creation of the legal health record (LHR) documentation, undertake the LHR definition project, and be responsible for its continued maintenance. Establishment of the stakeholder team should be the first step in the LHR definition process (Biedermann and Dolezel 2017, 430).

79. **a** Secondary data sources provide information that is not readily available from individual health records. Data taken from health records and entered into disease-oriented databases can help researchers determine the effectiveness of alternative treatment methods and monitor outcomes (Fahrenholz 2017c, 128).

80. **b** The National Committee on Vital and Health Statistics (NCVHS) has developed the initial efforts toward creating standardized data sets for use in different types of healthcare settings, including acute care, ambulatory care, long-term care, and home care (Fahrenholz 2017a, 62).

81. **a** Qualitative analysis is a review of the health record to ensure the adequacy of entries documenting the quality of care are present (Hunt 2017, 201).

82. **a** The continuity of care record (CCR) helps standardize clinical content for sharing between providers. A CCR allows documentation of care delivery from one healthcare experience to another (Sandefer 2020, 457).

83. **a** Regular reviews and updates of related policies and procedures to ensure the organization is always in compliance with the latest rules and trends in the legal health records (LHRs) is part of the LHR maintenance plan (Biedermann and Dolezel 2017, 432).

84. **a**   Analysis is a review of the health record for completeness and accuracy. HIM personnel can remind providers to complete items in the record and to sign orders and progress (Reynolds and Morey 2020, 125).

85. **a**   Create a matrix that defines each document type in the legal health record and determines the medium in which each element will appear. Such a matrix could include a column indicating the transition date of a particular document from the paper-based to the electronic environment. It is important that specific state guidelines are incorporated when a facility matrix is developed (Fahrenholz 2017c, 53).

86. **c**   The technology used to support the EHR can provide many enhancements over the paper record. Technology also presents the potential for weakening the integrity of the information. One such risk occurs with the copy-and-paste forward functionality present in many operating systems and software programs (Biedermann and Dolezel 2017, 449).

87. **b**   For elective hospital admissions, the patient or the admitting physician's office staff often provide administrative information and demographic data before the patient comes to the hospital. Alternatively, the patient may provide the information to the hospital's registration staff on the day of admission or through a secure page of the organization's website prior to admission. In the case of an unplanned admission, the patient or the patient's representative provides administrative information. A patient's name, age, and address would be considered administrative data (Johns 2015, 13).

88. **a**   The Healthcare Effectiveness Data and Information Set (HEDIS) is a set of standard performance measures designed to provide purchasers and consumers of healthcare with the information they need for comparing the performance of managed healthcare plans (Shaw and Carter 2019, 332).

89. **a**   Data quality management functions involve continuous improvement for data quality throughout an organization and include four key processes for data. These processes are application, collection, warehousing, and analysis. Analysis is the process of translating data into information utilized for an application (Shaw and Carter 2019, 79).

90. **c**   Applicable statutes of limitations, the time period in which a lawsuit may be filed, must be considered in establishing a retention schedule (Rinehart-Thompson 2017b, 195).

91. **b**   Only when copies of the personal health record (PHR) are used for treatment can they be considered part of the facilities' legal health record; however, the PHR does not replace the legal health record (Fahrenholz 2017d, 32–34).

92. **c**   Integrated delivery systems (IDS) typically have an enterprise master patient index (EMPI), which provides access to multiple repositories of information from overlapping patient populations that are maintained in separate information systems and databases (Sayles and Kavanaugh-Burke 2021, 157).

93. **a**   Organizations must address the final disposition of ePHI, hardware, and electronic media. There are four implementation specifications within this standard: disposal, media reuse, accountability, and data backup and storage (Biedermann and Dolezel 2017, 392).

94. **d**   Appropriate documentation of health record destruction must be maintained permanently no matter how the process is carried out. This documentation usually takes the form of a certificate of destruction (Fahrenholz 2017b, 108).

Domain 2 *Compliance with Access, Use, and Disclosure of Health Information*

95. **c** The concept of legal health records (LHRs) was created to describe the data, documents, reports, and information that comprise the formal business records of any healthcare organization that are to be utilized during legal proceedings (Biedermann and Dolezel 2017, 424).

96. **c** A secure patient portal does allow for the communication between the provider and the patient and is not just a site for patients to access information. This is part of the effort to engage patients in their care (Biedermann and Dolezel 2017, 458).

97. **a** Policies and procedures created by the covered entity or business associate to manage the use and disclosures of PHI should address the process for patient identification, including verification of the individual or personal representatives (Brinda and Watters 2020, 327).

98. **a** Under HIPAA, state law is considered more stringent if the law prohibits or restricts use or disclosure in circumstances under which such use or disclosure would be permitted under federal law (Brinda and Watters 2020, 330).

99. **c** Covered entities (healthcare organizations) are allowed to disclose protected health information for public health reporting purposes without an authorization or consent from the patient or family members. Since the whooping cough outbreak is a public health issue, it can be reported without authorization (Brinda and Watters 2020, 325).

100. **b** The Security Rule operationalizes the Privacy Rule and requires administrative safeguards such as policies and procedures to protect physical entities like information systems, buildings, and equipment (Brinda and Watters 2020, 319).

101. **d** If the data breach impacts less than 500 individuals, the covered entity or business associate must notify the secretary of the HHS annually; however, the notification must occur no later than 60 days after end of the calendar year in which the data breach occurred (Brinda and Watters 2020, 320).

102. **c** Timely response is an important part of the Privacy Rule. A covered entity must act on an individual's request for review of PHI no later than 30 days after the request is made, extending the response by no more than 30 days if within the 30 day time period it gives the reasons for the delay and the date by which it would respond (Rinehart-Thompson 2017, 245).

103. **c** Although the entity that created and maintains a patient's record is responsible for its physical integrity, and it is impossible to separate the information from the medium on which it resides, the information itself is the patient's (Rinehart-Thompson 2020, 60–61).

104. **b** HIPAA provides specific requirements regarding when protected health information can be used or disclosed with and without a signed authorization form by the patient. In this scenario a written authorization from the patient is needed in order to release the records to the daughter (Brinda and Watters 2020, 323).

105. **a** Compound authorizations combine the use and disclosure of PHI with other legal permissions such as consent for treatment, which is prohibited by the current HIPAA Privacy Rule (Brinda and Watters 2020, 324).

106. **d** Privileged communication is a legal concept designed to protect the confidentiality between two parties and is usually delineated by state law (Brodnik 2017a, 7).

107. **a** If physicians were to dictate information on patients they are treating in the facility, the disclosure of protected health information to the transcriptionists would be considered healthcare operations and, therefore, permitted under the HIPAA Privacy Rule. If physicians, who are separate covered entities, are dictating information on their private patients, however, it would be necessary for physicians to obtain a business associate agreement with the facility. It is permitted by the Privacy Rule for one covered entity to be a business associate of another covered entity (Thomason 2013, 26).

108. **b** Security audits are the mechanisms that record and examine activity in information systems. HIPAA does not specify what form of security audits must be used, how or how often they must be examined, or how long they must be retained (Brinda and Watters 2020, 334).

109. **c** The HIPAA Privacy Rule states that the covered entity must provide individuals with their information in the form that is requested by the individuals, if it is readily producible in the requested format. The covered entity can certainly decide, along with the individual, the easiest and least expensive way to provide the copies they request. Per the request of an individual, a covered entity must provide an electronic copy of any and all health information that the covered entity maintains electronically in a designated record set. If a covered entity does not maintain the entire designated record set electronically, there is not a requirement that the covered entity scan paper documents so the documents can be delivered electronically (Thomason 2013, 102).

110. **b** Original health records may be required by subpoena to be produced in person and the custodian of records is required to authenticate those records through testimony (Rinehart-Thompson 2017a, 59).

111. **a** The Professional Code of Ethics is based on ethical principles regarding privacy and confidentiality of patient information that have been an inherent part of the practice of medicine since the 4th century BC, when the Hippocratic Oath was created. Courts in various jurisdictions have concluded that a physician has a fiduciary duty to the patient to not disclose the patient's health and medical information (Theodos 2017, 14, 23).

112. **c** Patients (along with their next of kin or legal representatives) have the right to access their health records. However, health information management (HIM) professionals must validate the appropriateness of access. When a patient's next of kin or legal representative requests information belonging to the patient, HIM professionals should be familiar with state and federal laws regarding the right to access and who can authorize the use or disclosure of the information at issue (Fahrenholz 2017a, 45).

113. **c** The HIPAA Privacy Rule requires the covered entity to have business associate agreements in place with each business associate. This agreement must always include provisions regarding destruction or return of protected health information (PHI) upon termination of a business associate's services. Upon notice of the termination, the covered entity needs to contact the business associate and determine if the entity still retains any protected health information from, or created for, the covered entity. The PHI must be destroyed, returned to the covered entity, or transferred to another business associate. Once the PHI is transferred or destroyed, it is recommended that the covered entity obtain a certification from the business associate that either it has no protected health information, or all protected health information it had has been destroyed or returned to the covered entity (Thomason 2013, 18).

114. **c**   HITECH makes it easier for schools to receive student immunization records where state or other law requires it prior to student admission. HITECH permits CEs to disclose a child's immunization records (considered a public health activity) to a school with the oral consent of the parent or guardian. This contrasts with the previous written authorization requirement (Rinehart-Thompson 2017d, 246).

115. **a**   Data integrity means that data should be complete, accurate, consistent and up-to-date. With respect to data security, organizations must put protections in place so that no one may alter or dispose of data in a manner inconsistent with acceptable business and legal rules (Johns 2015, 211).

116. **c**   Individuals whose protected health information (PHI) has been breached must be provided with the following information: a description of what occurred (including date of breach and date that breach was discovered); the types of unsecured PHI that were involved (such as name, SSN, DOB, home address, and account number); steps that the individual may take to protect himself or herself; what the entity is doing to investigate, mitigate, and prevent future occurrences; contact information for the individual to ask questions and receive updates (AHIMA 2009; Rinehart-Thompson 2017d, 250–251).

117. **c**   The HIPAA Privacy Rule permits healthcare providers to access protected health information for treatment purposes. However, there is also a requirement that the covered entity provide reasonable safeguards to protect the information. These requirements are not easy to meet when the access is from an unsecured location, although policies, medical staff bylaws, confidentiality or other agreements, and a careful use of new technology can mitigate some risks (Thomason 2013, 46).

118. **b**   The HIPAA Privacy Rule allows communications to occur for treatment purposes. The preamble repeatedly states the intent of the rule is not to interfere with customary and necessary communications in the healthcare of the individual. Calling out a patient's name in a waiting room, or even on the facility's paging system, is considered an incidental disclosure and, therefore, allowed in the Privacy Rule (Thomason 2013, 37).

119. **c**   A firewall is a computer system or a combination of systems that provide a security barrier or support an access control policy between two networks or between a network and other traffic outside the network. This gatekeeper is physicially located between the routes of a public network like the Internet and those of a private network (Sayles and Kavanaugh-Burke 2021, 299).

120. **c**   Timely response is an important part of the Privacy Rule. A covered entity must act on an individual's request for review of PHI no later than 30 days after the request is made, extending the response by no more than 30 days if within the 30 day time period it gives the reasons for the delay and the date by which it would respond (Rinehart-Thompson 2017, 245).

121. **a**   It is generally agreed that Social Security numbers (SSNs) should not be used as patient identifiers. The Social Security Administration is adamant in its opposition to using the SSN for purposes other than those identified by law. AHIMA is in agreement on this issue due to privacy, confidentiality, and security issues related to the use of the SSN (Fahrenholz 2017b, 74).

122. **a**   The Privacy Rule states that an individual has a right of access to inspect and obtain a copy of his or her own PHI that is contained in a designated record set, such as a health record. The individual's right extends for as long as the PHI is maintained (Rinehart-Thompson 2017d, 243–244).

123. **b** Physical safeguards have to do with protecting the environment, including ensuring applicable doors have locks that are changed when needed and that fire, flood, and other natural disaster preparedness is in place (for example, fire alarms, sprinklers, smoke detectors, raised cabinets). Other physical controls include badging and escorting visitors and other typical security functions such as patrolling the premises, logging equipment in and out, and camera-monitoring key areas. HIPAA does not provide many specifics on physical facility controls but does require a facility security plan with the expectation that these matters will be addressed (Biedermann and Dolezel 2017, 390).

124. **c** One of the most fundamental terms in the Privacy Rule is PHI, defined by the rule as "individually identifiable health information that is transmitted by electronic media, maintained in electronic media, or transmitted or maintained in any other form or medium" (45 CFR 160.103). To meet the individually identifiable element of PHI, information must meet all three portions of a three-part test. (1) It must either identify the person or provide a reasonable basis to believe the person could be identified from the information given. (2) It must relate to one's past, present, or future physical or mental health condition; the provision of healthcare; or payment for the provision of healthcare. (3) It must be held or transmitted by a covered entity or its business associate (Rinehart-Thompson 2017c, 213).

125. **c** The HIPAA Security Rule requires covered entities to ensure the confidentiality, integrity, and availability of ePHI. The Security Rule contains provisions that require covered entities to adopt administrative, physical, and technical safeguards (Reynolds and Brodnik 2017a, 266–267).

126. **c** An EHR can provide highly effective access controls to meet the HIPAA Privacy Rule minimum necessary standard requirements. Role-based access controls are used where only specific classes of persons (for example, nurses) may access protected health information (Amatayakul 2017, 376–377).

127. **d** A firewall is a computer system or a combination of systems that provide a security barrier or support an access control policy between two networks or between a network and other traffic outside the network. This gatekeeper is physicially located between the routes of a public network like the Internet and those of a private network (Sayles and Kavanaugh-Burke 2021, 299).

128. **d** Option d categorically describes behavioral health, substance abuse, HIV/AIDS, genetic testing and adoption records, which are identified as highly sensitive information (Rinehart-Thompson 2020, 66).

129. **c** The 2013 HIPAA Omnibus Rule finalized regulations giving patients the right to request that their PHI not be disclosed to a health plan if they pay out of pocket in full for the services or items. A provider who accepts the payment and provides the service is compelled to abide by this request (Rinehart-Thompson 2017c, 220–221).

130. **a** An EHR can provide highly effective access controls to meet the HIPAA Privacy Rule minimum necessary standard requirements. Role-based access controls are used where only specific classes of persons may access protected health information. Context-based access controls add the dimensions that control not only class of persons but specific categories of information and under specific conditions for which access is permitted (Amatayakul 2017, 376–377).

131. **c** The facility access control standard requires covered entities to control and validate a person's access to a facility including visitor control (Biedermann and Dolezel 2017, 390–391).

132. **b**   Administrative safeguards are administrative actions such as policies and procedures and documentation retention to manage the selection, development, implementation, and maintenance of security measures to safeguard ePHI and manage the conduct of the covered entities or business associates' workforce (Biedermann and Dolezel 2017, 383).

133. **c**   Covered entities (CEs) are responsible for their workforce, which consists not only of employees but also volunteers, student interns, and trainees. Workforce members are not limited to those who receive wages from the CE (45 CFR 160.103(1); Rinehart-Thompson 2017c, 211).

134. **b**   Confidentiality is a legal ethical concept that establishes the healthcare provider's responsibility for protecting health records and other personal and private information from unauthorized use or disclosure (Brodnik 2017a, 7–8).

135. **a**   When an individual who is at or above the age of majority becomes incapacitated, either permanently or temporarily, another person should be designated to make decisions for that individual including decisions about the use and disclosure of the individual's PHI. Whoever serves as the incompetent adult's personal representative should, at minimum, hold the incompetent adult's durable power of attorney (DPOA) or durable power of attorney for healthcare decisions (DPOA-HCD) (Brodnik 2017b, 342).

136. **c**   It is the responsibility of the treating provider, in this case the physician who will be performing the surgery, to obtain informed consent and it may not be delegated to some other person (Klaver 2017c, 141).

137. **b**   The HIPAA Privacy Rule states that protected health information used for purposes of treatment, payment, or healthcare operations does not require patient authorization to allow providers access, use, or disclosure. However, only the minimum necessary information needed to satisfy the specified purpose can be used or disclosed (Rinehart-Thompson 2017c, 216–217).

138. **b**   The security audit process should include triggers that identify the need for a closer inspection. A trigger is a flag that notifies the organization of a possible security issue that needs investigation (Sayles and Kavanaugh-Burke 2021, 298).

139. **b**   A subpoena is a direct command that requires an individual or a representative of an organization to appear in court or to present an object to the court (Fahrenholz 2017b, 90–91).

140. **b**   HIPAA permits an individual to request that a covered entity make an amendment to PHI in a designated record set. However, the covered entity may deny the request if it determines that the PHI or the record was not created by the covered entity. In this scenario the history and physical was created by General Hospital. Mercy Hospital would be able to deny the request because they did not create the history and physical for this patient (Rinehart-Thompson 2018, 86).

141. **b**   Protecting the security and privacy of data in the database is called authorization management. Two of the important aspects of authorization management are user access control and usage monitoring (Rob and Coronel 2009; Amatayakul 2017, 376–377).

142. **c**   The Health Information Technology for Economic and Clinical Health Act (HITECH) shortened the time frame for an accounting of disclosures. Previously, an accounting had to include disclosures made during the previous six years. This has been shortened to disclosures made during the previous three years (Rinehart-Thompson 2018, 94).

143. **a**   The mental health professional can disclose information without an authorization from the patient in the following situations:

- The patient brings up the issue of the mental or emotional condition
- The health professional performs an examination under a court order
- Involuntary commitment proceedings
- A legal "duty to warn" an intended victim when a patient threatens to harm an identifiable victim(s)
- The mental health professional believes that the patient is likely to actually harm the individual(s) (Brodnik 2017b, 347–348).

144. **a**   Phishing is a scam by which an individual may receive an email that looks official but it is not. Its intent is to capture usernames, passwords, account numbers, and any other personal information. Users should be cautious in giving out confidential information such as passwords, credit card numbers, and social security numbers as many requests for this information received via email is a phishing scam (Sayles and Kavanaugh-Burke 2021, 303).

145. **b**   The HIPAA Privacy Rule allows individuals to decide whether they want to be listed in a facility directory when they are admitted to a facility. If the patient decides to be listed in the facility directory, the patient should be informed that only callers who know his or her name will be given any of this limited information. Covered entities generally do not, however, have to provide screening of visitors or calls for patients because such an activity is too difficult to manage with the number of employees and volunteers involved in the process of forwarding calls and directing visitors. If the covered entity agreed to the screening and could not meet the agreement, it could be considered a violation of this standard of the Privacy Rule (Thomason 2013, 105).

146. **d**   The Uniform Health Care Decisions Act suggests that decision-making priority for an individual's next-of-kin be as follows: spouse, adult child, parent, adult sibling, or if no one is available who is so related to the individual, authority may be granted to "an adult who exhibited special care and concern for the individual" (Klaver 2017c, 159–160).

147. **d**   Many state laws allow a minor to be treated as an adult for drug or alcohol dependency and sexually transmitted diseases or be given contraceptives and prenatal care without parental or legal guardian consent. This gives minors the right to treatment and access of their health records as a competent adult (Brodnik 2017b, 343–344).

148. **a**   Patients may sign in their names on a waiting room list, and if another patient sees it, that is considered an incidental disclosure. However, in determining the content of these sign-in lists, the healthcare provider must take reasonable precautions that the information is limited to the minimum necessary for the purpose (Thomason 2013, 38).

149. **c**   Generally, a hospital is liable to patients for the torts of its employees (including nurses and employed physicians) under the doctrine of *respondeat superior* (Latin for "let the master answer"). Also referred to as vicarious liability, under this doctrine the hospital holds itself out as responsible for the actions of its employees, provided that these individuals were acting within the scope of their employment or at the hospital's direction at the time they conducted the tortious activity in question (Rinehart-Thompson 2017b, 106–107).

150. **a** Employees in departments such as the business office, information systems, HIM, and infection control, who are not involved directly in patient care, will vary in their need to access patient information. The HIPAA "minimum necessary" principle must be applied to determine what access employees should legitimately have to PHI (45 CFR 164.502 [b]; Brodnik 2017b, 345).

151. **b** Reporting requirements mandate notification to the individual whose information was breached, and in the case of breaches of more than 500 individuals' information, to the media and the Secretary of Health and Human Services (Biedermann and Dolezel 2017, 401).

152. **b** The physician would not have access to records of a patient he or she is not treating unless the physician is performing designated healthcare operations such as research, peer review, or quality management. Otherwise the physician would need to have an authorization from the patient (Brodnik 2017b, 345–346).

153. **a** Encryption and destruction are the technologies and methodologies for rendering protected health information unusable, unreadable, or indecipherable to authorized individuals in order to prevent a potential breach of PHI (Biedermann and Dolezel 2017, 401).

154. **b** Job shadowing should be limited to areas where the likelihood of exposure to PHI is very limited, such as in administrative areas. There is a provision in the Privacy Rule that permits students and trainees to practice and improve their skills in the healthcare environment; however, the context of this provision appears to imply that the students are already enrolled in a healthcare field of study and that they are under the supervision of the covered entity. Most covered entities require students to be trained on confidentiality and other requirements of the Privacy Rule, and job shadowing activities do not appear to apply in this exception (Thomason 2013, 41).

155. **d** Redisclosure of health information is of significant concern to the healthcare industry. As such, the HIM professional must be alerted to state and federal statutes addressing this issue. A consent obtained by a hospital pursuant to the Privacy Rule in 45 CFR 164.506(a)(5) does not permit another hospital, healthcare provider, or clearinghouse to use or disclose information. However, the authorization content required in the Privacy Rule in 45 CFR 164.508(c)(1) must include a statement that the information disclosed pursuant to the authorization may be disclosed by the recipient and thus is no longer protected (Rinehart-Thompson 2017c, 231–232).

156. **d** One of the specifications found within the consent for use and disclosure of information should state that the individual has the right to revoke the consent in writing, except to the extent that the covered entity has already taken action based on the consent. In this situation, the facility acted in good faith based on the prior authorization and therefore the release is covered under the Privacy Act (Rinehart-Thompson 2017c, 223).

157. **a** Outcomes of quality improvement studies may be used to evaluate a physician's application for continued medical staff membership and privileges to practice. These studies are usually conducted as part of the hospital's QI activities. These review activities are considered confidential and protected from disclosure (Shaw and Carter 2019, 392–393).

158. **c** Employers who may or may not be HIPAA-covered healthcare organizations may request patient information for a number of reasons, including family medical leave certification, return to work certification for work-related injuries, and information for company physicians. Patient authorization is required for such disclosures, except in some states the patient's employer, employer's insurer, and employer's and employee's attorneys do not need patient authorization to obtain health information for workers' compensation purposes (Brodnik 2017b, 345).

159. **a**   News media personnel (and others) may have an interest in obtaining information about a public figure or celebrity who is being treated or about individuals involved in events that have cast them in the public eye. However, the media is not exempt from the restrictions imposed by the HIPAA facility directory requirement, and it is prudent for a healthcare organization to exercise even greater restraint than that mandated by the facility directory requirement with respect to the media. Parents of adult children and attorneys also need an authorization to receive patient records. A hospital may disclose health information to law enforcement when the suspected criminal conduct has resulted in a death (Brodnik 2017b, 365).

160. **c**   The maintenance of policies and procedures implemented to comply with the Security Rule must be retained for six years from the date of its creation or the date when it was last in effect, whichever is later (Reynolds and Brodnik 2017a, 278–279).

161. **d**   The implementation of the Health Insurance Portability and Accountability Act (HIPAA) Privacy Rule in 2003 established a consistent set of privacy and security rules. The Privacy Rule states that protected health information used for treatment, payment, or healthcare operations does not require patient authorization to allow providers access, use, or disclosure. However, only the minimum necessary information needed to satisfy the specified purpose can be used or disclosed. The release of information for purposes unrelated to treatment, payment, or healthcare operations still requires the patient's written authorization (Fahrenholz 2017a, 45–46).

162. **b**   A notice of privacy practices must be available at the site where the individual is treated and must be posted in a prominent place where the patient can be reasonably expected to read it (Rinehart-Thompson 2017c, 219).

163. **a**   The legal hold requires special, tracked handling of patient records to ensure no changes can be made in a record involved in litigation. This is common in the paper record environments to substantiate the integrity of the record and less common in the electronic environment where audit logs are the standard. Record managers need to address the use of legal hold for patient records in any information mode or medium (Biedermann and Dolezel 2017, 444–445).

164. **c**   Per HIPAA, covered entities may require individuals to make their access requests in writing if it has informed them of this requirement. A covered entity must act on an individual's request within 30 days, and may extend the response just once by no more than 30 days as long as it responds within the initial 30-day window and gives the reason for the delay and a date by which it will respond (Rinehart-Thompson 2018, 87).

165. **c**   There are certain circumstances where the minimum necessary requirement does not apply, such as to healthcare providers for treatment; to the individual or his or her personal representative; pursuant to the individual's authorization to the Secretary of the HHS for investigations, compliance review, or enforcement; as required by law; or to meet other Privacy Rule compliance requirements (Rinehart-Thompson 2017c, 234).

166. **c**   The Confidentiality of Alcohol and Drug Abuse Patient Records Rule is a federal rule that applies to information created for patients treated in a federally assisted drug or alcohol abuse program and specifically protects the identity, diagnosis, prognosis, or treatment of these patients. The rule generally prohibits redisclosure of health information related to this treatment except as needed in a medical emergency or when authorized by an appropriate court order or the patient's authorization (Rinehart-Thompson 2020, 66).

167. **d**   Because incident reports contain facts, hospitals strive to protect their confidentiality. To ensure incident report confidentiality, no copies should be made and the original must not be filed in the health record nor removed from the files in the department responsible for maintaining them, typically risk management or QI. Also no reference to the completion of an incident report should be made in the health record. Such a reference would likely render the incident report discoverable because it is mentioned in a document that is discoverable in legal proceedings (Rinehart-Thompson 2020, 68–69).

168. **c**   No authorization is needed to use or disclose PHI for public health activities. Some health records contain information that is important to the public welfare. Such information must be reported to the state's public health service to ensure public safety (Brinda and Watters 2020, 325).

169. **b**   A significant part of the administrative simplification process is the creation of standards for the electronic transmission of data (Rinehart-Thompson 2017c, 207).

170. **d**   The key to defining PHI is that it requires the information to either identify an individual or provide a reasonable basis to believe the person could be identified from the information given. In this situation, the information relates to a patient's health condition and could identify the patient (Rinehart-Thompson 2017c, 214).

171. **c**   Access control requires the implementation of technical policies and procedures for electronic information systems that maintain electronic protected health information (ePHI) to allow access only to those persons or software programs that have been granted access rights as specified in the administrative safeguards. There are four implementation specifications with this standard, one of which includes emergency access procedures, which are procedures established to grant individuals access to ePHI in an emergency (Reynolds and Brodnik 2017a, 276–277).

172. **b**   The Breach Notification Rule requires covered entities and business associates to establish policies and procedures to investigate an authorized use or disclosure of PHI to determine if a breach occurred, conclude the investigation, and to notify affected individuals and the Secretary of HHS within 60 days of date of discovery of the breach (Brinda and Watters 2020, 320).

173. **c**   The three methods of two-factor authentication are something you know, such as a password or PIN; something you have, such as an ATM card, token, or swipe/smart card; and something you are, such as a biometric fingerprint, voice scan, iris, or retinal scan (Sayles and Kavanaugh-Burke 2021, 295-296).

174. **b**   Pursuant to the Privacy Rule, the hospital may disclose health information to law enforcement officials without authorization for law enforcement purposes for certain situations, including situations involving a crime victim. Disclosure is made in response to law enforcement officials' request for such information about an individual who is, or is suspected to be, a victim of a crime (Brinda and Watters 2020, 325).

175. **a**   Training in HIPAA policies and procedures regarding PHI is required for all workforce members to carry out their job functions appropriately. The training should be ongoing and documented for each employee (Biedermann and Dolezel 2017, 371).

176. **a**   Legislation gives a patient the right to obtain an accounting of disclosures of PHI made by the covered entity in the six years or less prior to the request date. Mandatory public health reporting is not considered part of a covered entities' operations. As a result, these disclosures must be included in an accounting of disclosures (Rinehart-Thompson 2017d, 247–248).

Domain 3 *Data Analytics and Informatics*

177. **a**   An encoder is used to increase the accuracy and efficiency of the coding process. Encoders promote accuracy as well as consistency in the coding of diagnoses and procedures (Amatayakul 2017, 292).

178. **b**   The average turnaround time was calculated by dividing the total response days attributed to the volume of routine requests that were responded to within the reporting period by the volume of routine requests responded to. The calculation is: $(200 \times 3) + (100 \times 5) + (50 \times 8) + (50 \times 10)/400 = 5$ days (Oachs 2020, 778).

179. **a**   Productivity standards should be aligned with the organization's mission and goals of the organization (Oachs 2020, 772).

180. **a**   The provenance (or source) of data is considered a form of administrative metadata. The other choices relate to metadata, but are not illustrative of any given form of metadata (Amatayakul 2020, 437–438).

181. **b**   The yes or no question as to whether mother smoked during pregnancy would be nominal data with numbers assigned to them for a calculation. The baby's birth weight is a ratio or scale data because it is a defined unit of measure. The APGAR scores represent ordinal data because the order of the numbers is meaningful (White 2020a, 196–197).

182. **d**   Observing how an EHR is used, such as whether comment fields are frequently used when structured data should have been used or first choice in a list is selected over a choice that is more specific, is the best way to determine root cause of poor quality of data. Other choices may be indicators of poor quality but also include other factors as well (Amatayakul 2020, 439).

183. **c**   Simple linear regression (SLR) is another type of statistical inference that not only measures the strength of the relationship between two variables, but also estimates a functional relationship between them. SLR may be used when one of the two variables of interest is dependent on the other (White 2020b, 517).

184. **b**   Identification of need is one phase of the modern systems development life cycle (SDLC). One of the components of this phase is to identify budgeting, scheduling, and personnel constraints (Amatayakul 2017, 46).

185. **a**   System customization enables an organization to make adjustments to how software is used and displayed. Adjusting decision support rules (such as turning them off, or narrowing the specifications for a given rule) are made possible by vendor-supplied tools that do not impact the underlying software (Amatayakul 2020, 427).

186. **b**   Stewardship refers to taking care of something you own or have been entrusted with. Given the choices here, EHR data stewardship is exemplified by ensuring proper data entry; contributing to design and maintaining data in an information system are beyond the requirements of the average healthcare professional and not sharing data appropriately is actually not good data stewardship (Amatayakul 2020, 438–439).

187. **a**   Agreeing on standards and how they are to be implemented for successful mapping between systems is an important part of governance (Lee-Eichenwald 2020, 387).

188. **d** ASCX12 refers to standards adopted for electronic data interchange. In order for transmission of healthcare data between a provider and payer, both parties must adhere to these standards (Sayles and Kavanaugh-Burke 2021, 282).

189. **a** Benchmarking is the systematic comparison of the products, services, and outcomes of an organization with those of a similar organization. Benchmarking comparisons also can be made using regional and national standards or some combination (Shaw and Carter 2019, 42).

190. **b** The physical data model shows how the data are physically stored within the database. The users are not involved with this level of the database because of its technical complexity (Sayles and Kavanaugh-Burke 2021, 47).

191. **c** Reliability is frequently checked by having more than one person abstract data for the same case. The results are then compared to identify any discrepancies. This is called an interrater reliability method of checking. Several different people may be used to do the checking. In the cancer registry, physician members of the cancer committee are called on to check the reliability of the data (Houser 2020, 571).

192. **c** Work sampling is a technique of work measurement that involves using statistical probability (determined through random sample observations) to characterize the performance of the department and its work (functional) units (Oachs 2020, 775).

193. **c** In addition to bar codes on medical record documents, optical character recognition (OCR) may be available to enhance the accuracy of indexing features on forms (Lee-Eichenwald 2020, 363).

194. **b** In the HIPAA Security Rule, one of the technical safeguards standards is access control. This includes automatic log-off, which ensures electronics processes that terminate an electronic session after a predetermined time of inactivity (Reynolds and Brodnik 2017a, 277).

195. **b** Structured query language (SQL) defines data elements, manipulates data, and controls access (Sayles and Kavanaugh-Burke 2021, 40).

196. **b** In data mining, the analyst performs exploratory data analysis to determine trends and identify patterns in the data set (White 2020b, 520).

197. **d** The Digital Imaging and Communications in Medicine (DICOM) standard supports retrieval of information from imaging devices and equipment to diagnostic and review workstations as well as short-term and long-term storage systems (Amatayakul 2017, 404–405).

198. **c** Within healthcare, standard protocols that support communication between nonintegrated applications are often referred to as messaging standards, also called interoperability standards or data exchange standards. Messaging standards provide the tools to map proprietary formats to one another and more easily accomplish the exchange of data (Amatayakul 2017, 400–401).

199. **d** A scatter diagram is a data analysis tool used to plot points of two variables suspected of being related to each other in some way (Oachs 2020, 789).

200. **d** A web portal is a single point of personalized access (an entryway) through which to find and deliver information (content), applications, and services. Web portals began in the consumer market as an integration strategy rather than a solution. Portals offered users of the large, public Internet service provider websites, fast, centralized access (via a web browser) to an array of Internet services and information found on those websites (Lee-Eichenwald 2020, 365).

201. **c** Enterprise master patient indexes (EMPIs) provide access to multiple repositories of information from overlapping patient populations that are maintained in separate systems and databases. This occurs through an indexing scheme to all unique patient identification numbers and information in all the organizations' databases. As such, EMPIs become the cornerstones of healthcare system integration projects (Reynolds and Morey 2020, 132).

202. **b** Quantity standards (also called productivity standards) and quality standards (also known as service standards) are generally used by managers to monitor individual employee performance and the performance of a functional unit or the department as a whole. To properly communicate performance standards, managers need to make the distinction between quantitative and qualitative standards and identify examples of each for the HIS functions. In the scenario, transcribing 1,500 lines per day is identifying the quantity of work rather than how well the work is being performed so it is a quantity standard (Oachs 2020, 773).

203. **a** If an EHR is to provide clinical decision support it requires structured data (Sayles and Kavanaugh Burke 2021, 216-217).

204. **a** Preventive controls are front-end processes that guide work in such a way that input and process variations are minimized. Simple things such as standard operating procedures, edits on data entered into computer-based systems, and training processes are ways to reduce the potential for error by using preventive controls (Oachs 2020, 777).

205. **c** A data flow diagram is a diagram of how data flows in the database. The data flow diagram is a good way to show management and other nontechnical users the system design (Sayles and Kavanaugh-Burke 2021, 48).

206. **a** Typically, provider-based portal uses include requesting prescription renewal, scheduling appointments, and asking questions of providers via secure messaging. Patients may also pay bills online or securely view all or portions of the electronic health record, such as current medical conditions, medications, allergies, and test results. Patients would not be able to edit their health record information (Lee-Eichenwald 2020, 365).

207. **a** A pie chart is an easily understood chart in which the sizes of the slices of the pie show the proportional contribution of each part. Pie charts can be used to show the component parts of a single group or variable and are intended for interval or ratio data (Marc 2020, 537).

208. **a** Many organizations have discovered that paying insufficient attention to workflow and process improvement in the EHR planning stages can lead to serious negative outcomes. This is the time to map current processes (Amatayakul 2019, 126-127).

209. **a** The HIM department can plan focused reviews based on specific problem areas after the initial baseline review has been completed. This would be called a focused coding review (Schraffenberger and Kuehn 2011, 314–315).

210. **a** MPI management must include continuous maintenance and correction of data integrity problems. Ongoing education of registration and scheduling staff is critical to maintaining low creation rates for duplicates, overlays, and other EMPI data integrity problems (Reynolds and Morey 2020, 132–133).

211. **c** The centralized HIE model stores patient records in a single database built to allow queries into the system. This model tends to return results quicker than other models (Lee-Eichenwald 2020, 387–388).

212. **c** Health Level 7 (HL7) is a nonprofit organization that develops standards for interoperability of health information technology (Fahrenholz 2017a, 63).

213. **a** Extranets are networks that connect a given organization to its customers and business partners or suppliers (business associates in healthcare). Although extranets send information over public networks, requiring a greater level of security, access to them is still restricted to the services and persons authorized (Lee-Eichenwald 2020, 366).

214. **c** Part of a coding compliance plan is to identify areas of risk through audits and monitoring. Selecting the types of cases to review is also important. Examples of various case selection possibilities include medical and surgical MS-DRSs by high dollar and volume. Auditing cases with infrequent diagnosis and procedure codes, low dollar and low volume, and low admission diagnoses would not be as suitable (Hunt and Kirk 2020, 296).

215. **b** To calculate the case mix index from the volume of cases from MS-DRG calculate the weighted average MS-DRG weight by completing these steps: (1) Multiply the number of discharges in each MS-DRG by the relative weight of that MS-DRG; (2) Sum the relative weights from step 1; (3) Sum the number of discharges in the MS-DRGs chosen to be evaluated; (4) Divide the total relative weights from step 2 by the total number of discharges from step 3.

    Step 1:

    $3.9994 \times 100 = 399.94$

    $2.2838 \times 52 = 118.7576$

    $1.8807 \times 36 = 67.7052$

    Step 2:

    $3.9994 + 118.7576 + 67.7052 = 586.4028$

    Step 3:

    $100 + 52 + 36 = 188$

    Step 4:

    $586.4028 \div 188 = \mathbf{3.1192}$

    (White 2021, 164)

216. **b** Interoperability is often described in levels. The NCVHS has identified three levels: basic, functional, and semantic. Basic interoperability relates to the ability to successfully transmit and receive data from one computer to another. Functional interoperability refers to sending messages between computers with a shared understanding of the structure and format of the message. The use of clinical terminologies in EHRs to provide standardized data is essential to achieving semantic interoperability (Palkie 2020a, 157).

217. **a** Bar graphs are used to display data from one or more variables. The bars may be drawn vertically or horizontally. Bar charts are used for nominal or ordinal variables. In this case, you would be displaying the average length of stay by service and then within each service have a bar for each gender (White 2020a, 209).

218. **b** Requirements refer to those elements that must exist; hence, the features and functions that must be in an information system should be included in a requirements specification (among other things) (Amatayakul 2020, 423).

219. **c** The result management application enables the results of diagnostic studies to be compared and displayed with other data (Amatayakul 2017, 14).

220. **c** Sampling is used when examining the entire population is either too time consuming or too expensive. A sample is the subset of the population or universe. The universe is the set of all units that are eligible to be sampled. A listing of all of the subjects in the universe is called the sampling frame. The universe in a sampling plan may be patients, physicians, health records, or any other unit of analysis that is studied. In this case, the sample unit is the claim (White 2021, 148).

221. **a** Demographic data includes basic factual details about the individual patient. The main purpose of collecting demographic data is to confirm the patients' identity. Hospitals and other healthcare–related organizations use the demographic data collected from patients as the basis of statistical records, research, and resource planning (Fahrenholz 2017b, 74).

222. **d** Once a current process has been mapped, it is important to validate that map is complete and accurate (Amatayakul 2017, 136).

223. **b** Reflections of original data, often referred to generally as image data, include document images, unstructured text data, video, audio, vectors, and diagnostic images (Amatayakul 2017, 285).

224. **a** The acquisition phase of the modern systems development life cycle (SDLC), one of the steps is to negotiate the contract (Amatakayul 2017, 48).

225. **a** A data administrator focuses on understanding interrelationships among data in order to prepare a logical design for a database. A database administrator is an information technology specialist in database implementation and maintenance. Data governance managers are, typically, users of databases. Data technologist is not a commonly used job title, but it may be one who manages metadata (Amatayakul 2020, 414).

226. **d** Secondary analysis is the analysis of the original work of others. In secondary analysis, researchers reanalyze original data by combining data sets to answer new questions or by using more sophisticated statistical techniques. The work of others created the MEDPAR file (Houser 2020, 563).

227. **b** A data model is an important part of describing how data will be processed. It has other uses as well, but the model itself does not define the data, show how it is displayed, or list attributes. Most of these functions are performed by a data dictionary (Amatayakul 2020, 437).

228. **a** Auditing structured data can reveal a number of potential data quality issues, such as when all choices for a structured field are the same, when a structured field is often empty. Comparing data in the EHR to dictated documents is an extremely time-consuming process and would only be used after auditing structured data; there are virtually no established norms for quality specific to a given data element, and determining an acceptable error rate is not an assessment of quality (Amatayakul 2020, 439).

229. **a** Clinical pathways are a tool designed to coordinate multidisciplinary care planning for specific diagnoses and treatments (O'Dell 2020, 631-632).

230. **d** Dashboards is a display of process measures to help leaders follow progress to assist with strategic planning. The dashboard provides the status on key measures (Sayles and Kavanaugh-Burke 2021, 328).

231. **b** Quantity standards (also called productivity standards) and quality standards (also known as service standards) are generally used by managers to monitor individual employee performance and the performance of a functional unit or the department as a whole. To properly communicate performance standards, managers need to make the distinction between quantitative and qualitative standards and identify examples of each for the HIS functions. In the scenario, completing five birth certificates per hour is identifying the quantity of work rather than how well the work is being performed so it is a quantity standard (Oachs 2020, 773).

232. **c** Control charts can be used to measure key processes over time. Using a control chart focuses attention on any variation in a process (Shaw and Carter 2019, 88–89).

233. **a** Association rule learning is a type of data mining identifies interesting relationships between two concepts in the database. For example, it may identify that patients who are treated with drug A have a better outcome than patients who are treated with drug B (Sayles and Kavanaugh-Burke 2021, 53).

234. **a** Descriptive analytics use a group of statistical techniques to describe data such as means, frequency distributions, and is used to describe the characteristics of a specific group or population (Sayles and Kavanaugh-Burke 2021, 36).

235. **c** This process involves the use of standardized terminologies, such as SNOMED-CT, to provide clarity, consistency, and appropriate meaning in HIE (Sayles and Kavanaugh-Burke 2021, 253).

236. **a** Clinical messaging is the function of electronically delivering data and automating the workflow around the management of clinical data. Clinical messages can use e-mail, portals, virtual private networks, and other means to provide the secure means of communication needed for patient information. These messages are shared in such a way as to protect the privacy of the patient (Sayles and Kavanaugh-Burke 2021, 209).

237. **a** The staffing level is determined by dividing the number of images by the expected productivity. An FTE is the total number of workers, including part-time, in an area as the equivalent of full-time positions. Divide 48,000 by maximum standard work per hour for each function then add up the calculated hours for each function and divide by 8 (White 2020a, 157).

238. **b** A database is an organized collection of data, text, references, or pictures in a standardized format, typically stored in a computer system for multiple applications. The databased can used to create reports, download into spreadsheets, trending and more (Sayles and Kavanaugh-Burke 2021, 328).

239. **c** CAC may be performed while the patient is still in the hospital and then updated after discharge. Doing so speeds up the coding turnaround time and improves efficiency because coding rules are applied consistently, and error rates are reduced (Sayles and Kavanaugh-Burke 2021, 129).

240. **c** Personal health records electronically populate elements or subsets of protected health information (PHI) from provider organization databases into the electronic records of authorized patients, their families, other providers, and sometimes health payers and employers. A range of people and groups maintain the records, including the patients, their families, and other providers (Reynolds and Morey 2020, 117).

241. **a** Performance standards are often developed for the key functions of the job and set the quantity and quality for each job function (LeBlanc 2020, 700).

242. **d** The range is the simplest measure of spread. It is the difference between the smallest and largest values in a frequency distribution:

$$\text{Range} = x_{max} - x_{min}$$

For this scenario, the range is 1 to 29 (29 − 1) or 28 (White 2020a, 182).

243. **a** Predictive modeling applies statistical techniques to determine the likelihood of certain events occurring together (White 2021, 10).

244. **d** Natural language queries use common words to tell the database which data are needed (Sayles and Kavanaugh-Burke 2021, 40).

245. **c** Hospital-acquired (nosocomial) infection rates may be calculated for the entire hospital or for a specific unit in the hospital. They also may be calculated for the specific types of infections. Ideally, the hospital should strive for an infection rate of 0.0 percent. The formula for calculating the hospital-acquired, or nosocomial, infection rate is: Total number of hospital-acquired infections for a given period/Total number of discharges, including deaths, for the same period × 100 (Edgerton 2020, 490).

246. **a** Auditing a random selection of EHR documentation would be the best approach for avoiding selection bias and in determining how the copy function is being used (Houser 2020, 562).

247. **b** A histogram is used to display a frequency distribution. It is different from a bar graph in that a bar graph is used to display data that fall into groups or categories (nominal or ordinal data) when the categories are noncontinuous or discrete (Marc 2020, 538).

248. **b** The one-to-many relationship exists when one instance of an entity is associated with many instances of another entity. If a physician may be linked to many patients and patients may only be related to one physician, this is an example of a one-to-many relationship (Sayles and Kavanaugh-Burke 2021, 47-48).

249. **c** Scheduling systems are used to control the use of resources throughout the healthcare facility. These resources can include staff, equipment, rooms, and more. Scheduling systems may be centralized or independent (Sayles and Kavanaugh-Burke 2021, 160).

250. **d** Health information blocking occurs when persons or entities knowingly and unreasonably interfere with the exchange or use of electronic health information. Blocking stems from healthcare providers or HIT vendors protecting their own proprietary and business interests above the interests of the patient and healthcare improvement. These efforts actively impede the progress sought by the concept of EHRs and health information exchange (Sayles and Kavanaugh-Burke 2021, 204).

251. **c** A line plot is used for two main purposes: (1) to present trends or patterns in the number of occurrences between groups or (2) to present trends or patterns in the mean of a variable between groups. Typically, the change of a variable over time is compared. In this case, the trend that can be summarized by this line plot is that the LOS for Hospital B has increased and for Hospital a has decreased since the 1st quarter (Marc 2020, 537).

252. **b** A method that has been developed for presenting a variety of data on a single display in an easy-to-read format is called a dashboard (Marc 2020, 538).

253. **a** Nursing documentation traditionally includes medication administration record. These records are maintained by nursing staff for all patients and include medication given, time, form of administration, and dose and strength (Reynolds and Morey 2020, 114).

254. **d** Classification analysis is a method of identifying important information about the data in the database by grouping data much like grouping diagnoses and procedures Sayles and Kavanaugh-Burke 2021, 53).

255. **a** A clinical data repository is a centralized database that captures, sorts, and processes patient data and then sends it back to the user (Amatayakul 2017, 24).

256. **a** A disease index is a listing in diagnosis code number order for patients discharged from the facility during a particular time period. Each patient's diagnoses are converted from a verbal description to a numerical code, usually using a coding system such as the International Classification of Diseases (ICD) (Sharp and Madlock-Brown 2020, 178).

257. **d** For data that is presenting changes over time, the preferred presentation method is a line plot (Marc 2020, 537).

258. **d** Skewness is the horizontal stretching of a frequency distribution to one side or the other so that one tail is longer than the other. The direction of skewness is on the side of the long tail. Thus, if the longer tail is on the right, the curve is skewed to the right. If the longer tail is on the left, the curve is skewed to the left (White 2020a, 186, 290).

259. **c** The hospital-acquired infection rate is $(4 \times 100)/57 = 400/57 = 7.0\%$. Hospital-acquired (nosocomial) infection rates may be calculated for the entire hospital. They also may be calculated for the specific types of infections. Ideally, the hospital should strive for an infection rate of 0.0 percent (Edgerton 2020, 490).

260. **a** The use of CPOE can lead to significant improvements in patient safety because of the reminders or alerts built into the system. Although alerts and reminders are useful, too many become frustrating to the physicians because they have to constantly stop their data entry to address the alerts and reminders (Sayles and Kavanaugh-Burke 2021, 209-210).

261. **a** Structural metadata is the process of acquiring, storing, manipulating, and displaying data. Data models, such as entity-relationship diagrams (ERD) and dataflow diagrams (DFD) are diagrammatical or graphic tools used to help program the system and to identify areas of inefficiency (Sayles and Kavanaugh-Burke 2021, 42).

262. **a** The decision support system (DSS) is an information system that gathers data from a variety of sources and assists in providing structure to the data by using various analytical models and visual tools in order to facilitate and improve the ultimate outcome in decision-making tasks associated with the nonroutine and nonrepetitive problems (Sayles and Kavanaugh-Burke 2021, 154).

263. **a** The population health component in an EHR is designed to capture and report healthcare data that are used for public health purposes. It allows the healthcare provider to report infectious diseases, immunizations, cancer, and other reportable conditions to public health officials. This reporting is required at the local, state, and national levels and includes infectious diseases. A population health system also can connect with public health officials to receive alerts regarding health issues (Sayles and Kavanaugh-Burke 2021, 211).

264. **b** The encoder is specialty software used by coders to select the appropriate code for the diagnosis(es) and procedure(s) supported by the health record. A grouper is a computer program that uses specific data elements to assign the diagnostic and procedural codes entered into the encoder into the appropriate Medicare severity diagnosis-related group (MS-DRG) or other diagnosis-related group (DRG) (Sayles and Kavanaugh-Burke 2021, 123).

265. **b** The federated architectural type has become more prevalent for health information organizations. There are two forms of this architecture. The consistent federated form is very similar to the consolidated architecture in which the data repository is partitioned but centrally managed. The consistent federated form, however, takes this one step further and physically separates the data but still offers centralized management. Essentially, this is much like an application service provider (ASP) or software as a service (SaaS) model of acquiring software (Amatayakul 2017, 417–418).

266. **c** The median is the midpoint of a frequency distribution and falls in the ordinal scale of measurement. It is the point at which 50 percent of the observations fall above and 50 percent fall below. If an odd number of observations is in the frequency distribution, the median is the middle number. In this data set, 8 is the middle number (White 2020a, 177).

267. **d** The proportionate mortality ratio (PMR) is a measure of mortality due to a specific cause for a specific time period. In the formula for calculating the PMR, the numerator is the number of deaths due to a specific disease for a specific time period, and the denominator is the number of deaths from all causes for the same time period. The proportionate mortality ratio for diabetes mellitus = 73,249/2,443,387 = 0.03 × 100 = 3.0% (AHIMA 2017, 192; Edgerton 2020, 476).

268. **c** A chart offers the advantage of seeing the general trend of data and comparing differences in data between groups or over time. However, the precise numeric values are more easily discerned when reading a table (Marc 2020, 529–530).

269. **b** Because there is no mandated unique patient identifier, ensuring that the HIE organization can identify the right patient as it seeks to exchange information is a process of identity matching (Amatayakul 2017, 419).

270. **c** If a particular medication were prescribed to the patient, the physician may not know that it would contraindicate the use of this certain drug because of the pre-existing allergy; the pharmacy information system (PIS) would alert the physician to this contraindication and suggestion another medication (Sayles and Kavanaugh-Burke 2021, 185).

271. **b** Health informatics must consider the development of standards for software to be used in the EHR and the exchange of data. Compatibility and interoperability, allowing different health information systems to work together within and across organizational boundaries in order to advance the effective delivery of healthcare for individuals and communities, are a key focus in health informatics (Biedermann and Dolezel 2017, 22).

272. **b** These documents should be followed during the testing process to ensure that the instructions in the documents are accurate (Sayles and Kavanaugh Burke 2021, 100).

273. **b** Slicing and dicing refers to the process of taking what is known at the highest level of understanding and working downward to identify the underlying causes for the high-level observation. A dashboard helps facilitate a greater understanding of financial, operational, and clinical processes to identify problems and successes (Marc 2020, 539).

274. **b** A boxplot displays the descriptive statistics of a continuous variable including the minimum, first quartile, medium, third quartile, maximum, and potential outlier values. The line that makes the bottom of the box represents the value for the first quartile; the first quartile of a dataset is used to represent the 25th percentile of numeric data. In other words, the number representing the first quartile can be interpreted as a value at which 25 percent of the numbers in the dataset have a value equal to or less than that value. The line that makes the top of the box represents the value for the third quartile. The third quartile represents the 75th percentile. The number representing the third quartile is interpreted as a value at which 75 percent of the numbers in the dataset have a value equal to or less than that value. If there are dots above and below the boxes, these dots represent potential outliers. An outlier is a value that is distant from other values. The graph shows the widest range of values in hospital A as demonstrated by the difference between the lowest and upper whiskers. Also, hospital A displays with the highest median wait time (Marc 2020, 537).

275. **b** A secure patient portal does allow for the communication between the provider and the patient and is not just a site for patients to access information. This is part of the effort to engage patients in their care. Patient are able to complete appointment scheduling through a patient portal (Biedermann and Dolezel 2017, 458).

276. **c** For whatever architecture an HIE organization may have, there needs to be a way to identify participants, which may include individual providers, representatives of payer organizations, and patients or consumers, as well as organizational entities and their information systems. This service is called registry and directory (Amatayakul 2017, 418–419).

277. **c** Algorithms are used by organizations to determine the probability of a duplicate in order to identify potential duplicate MPI entries (Reynolds and Morey 2020, 132-133).

278. **d** Prescriptive analytics uses information generated from descriptive and prescriptive analytics and modeling to determine a strategy for the best outcome and/or to suggest a course of action to solve a problem (Sayles and Kavanaugh-Burke 2021, 36).

279. **c** Data analytics is the science of examining raw data with the purpose of drawing conclusions about that information. This information can then be used to make business decisions concerning which serves to provide and how to improve patient care (Sayles and Kavanaugh-Burke 2021, 8-9).

280. **b** In data mining, the analyst performs exploratory data analysis to determine trends and identify patterns in the data set. Data mining is sometimes referred to as knowledge discovery (White 2020b, 520).

281. **b** Practice management systems are used by physician practices. Scheduling, patient accounting, patient collections, claims submission, appointment scheduling, human resources, and other functions all are built into this single information system (Sayles and Kavanaugh-Burke 2021, 160).

282. **c** Histograms are used to present the distribution of numeric data. The numeric variable is broken down into groups based on specific ranges of values to establish the widths of each bar in a histogram. The height of each bar represents the frequency or density of each of the binned groups. The distribution can be described as normally distributed when the pattern follows a bell-shaped pattern (Marc 2020, 538).

283. **d**   The CDI information system assists HIM and CDI staff in the physician query process by facilitating communication between the coding professional and the physician (Sayles and Kavanaugh-Burke 2021, 139).

284. **a**   Preventive controls are front end processes that guide work in such a way that input and process variations are minimized. In the list of possible answers, only adding an edit occurs at the front end to prevent the error from happening. The reporting and audit are after the error occurred and considered feedback controls (Oachs 2020, 777).

285. **a**   A standard is a scientifically based statement of expected behavior against which structures, processes, and outcomes can be measured. Standards are important to the electronic health record (EHR) because they streamline the communication method that allows information systems to speak to each other and for data to be stored using the same formats, language, and terms to describe and execute functions (Sayles and Kavanaugh-Burke 2021, 318).

286. **a**   When developing the data elements that go into a database, the fields should be normalized. Normalization is breaking the data elements into the level of detail desired by the facility. For example, last name and first name should be in separate fields as should city, state, and zip code (Sayles and Kavanaugh-Burke 2021, 49).

287. **a**   The Office of the National Coordinator (ONC) has been driving the escalation of technology through its National Strategic Framework requirement of mandating the implementation of EHRs and currently toward the acceleration of health information exchange (HIE) (Palkie 2020b, 312).

288. **b**   Consumer health informatics is a field devoted to informatics from multiple consumer or patient views and includes patient-focused informatics, health literacy, and consumer education, with a focus on information structures and processes that empower consumers to manage their own health (AMIA n.d.; Sandefer 2020, 447).

289. **b**   The first step in statistical hypothesis testing is defining the null and alternative hypotheses. The null hypothesis is the status quo. In this example the readmission rates are equal would be the null hypothesis showing no relationship between the two hospitals (White 2021, 76).

290. **d**   Data about patients can be extracted from individual health records and combined as aggregate data. Aggregate data are used to develop information about groups of patients. In this case, the fact that 50 percent of patients treated at our facilities have Medicare as their primary payer is data about patients combined together, so it is aggregate data (Sharp and Madlock-Brown 2020, 176).

291. **d**   The probability of making a Type I error based on a particular set of data is called the p-value (White 2020b, 504).

292. **b**   To enhance retrieval of scanned documents, some form of indexing needs to take place in order to organize the documents. Ideally, each form that is scanned or otherwise created should have a bar code or some other forms recognition feature, or features, associated with it (Amatayakul 2017, 285).

293. **a**   Diagnostic analytics helps a healthcare organization determine why something happened. Diagnostic analytics tools such as dashboards and data mining are performed (Sayles and Kavanaugh-Burke 2021, 36).

294. **b**   LOINC is set of terminology standards that provide a standard set of universal names and codes for identifying individual laboratory and clinical results (Palkie 2020a, 159).

295. **c**   If the sample has extreme values on either the high or low end of the scale, then the median may be the better choice for describing the center of the distribution. The median is less influenced by outliers (White 2020b, 509).

Domain 4   *Revenue Cycle Management*

296. **a**   A healthcare-associated infection (HAI) is an infection occurring in a patient in a hospital or healthcare setting in whom the infection was not present or incubating at the time of admission, or it is the remainder of an infection acquired during a previous admission (Shaw and Carter 2019, 177).

297. **a**   Revenue integrity is performing revenue cycle duties to obtain operational efficiency, compliance adherence, and legitimate reimbursement. A claim that is clean, complete, and compliant meets the goals of revenue integrity (Casto and White 2021, 9-10).

298. **d**   Medicare allows for 100 skilled days of care per calendar year (Hazelwood 2020, 213-214).

299. **a**   Fee-for-service reimbursement is based on the principle that there is a charge for each service rendered by a provider (Hazelwood 2020, 225).

300. **c**   The total out-of-pocket patient responsibility for this inpatient stay is $6,820. The patient must pay the deductible for the benefit period which is $1,364. Days 1–60 are covered by deductible. The remaining 16 days of care are charged at $341 per day, or $5,456. (March 1–March 31 is 31 days of care; April 1–April 30 is 30 days of care; May 1–May 15 is 15 days of care for a total of 76 days of care). The total charge for this hospital stay is $6,820 ($5,456 + $1,364) (Hazelwood 2020, 213).

301. **a**   The correct answers is "Y=Yes" as the condition is present on admission. When the patient was admitted from observation, the hip fracture was present (Hazelwood 2020, 230–231).

302. **d**   Many organizations create policies to follow reasonable registration procedures and occur after medical screening (Handlon 2020, 246).

303. **c**   The scrubber reviews the claim for errors using predetermined criteria prior to sending to the payer for payment (Handlon 2020, 262).

304. **a**   Global payments are lump-sum payments for an entire event. These may be distributed among different physicians or between physicians and facilities. For many radiological procedures, the physician is paid for the professional component of the procedure while the facility is paid for the technical component (supplies, technician, equipment, and the like). Unbundled payments should not occur, and fee-for-service is payment for each individual component of a service and not a lump sum (Hazelwood 2020, 226–227).

305. **a**   The formula for measuring the days in total discharged, not final billed is calculated with a numerator of gross dollars in discharged not filled billed and a denominator of average daily gross patient service revenue (Handlon 2020, 269).

306. **d**   Determinations of medical necessity must reflect the efficient and cost-effective application of patient care including, but not limited to, diagnostic testing, therapies (including activity restriction, after-care instructions, and prescriptions), disability ratings, rehabilitating an illness, injury, disease or its associated symptoms, impairments or functional limitations, procedures, psychiatric care, levels of hospital care, extended care, long-term care, hospice care, and home healthcare (Handlon 2020, 248).

307. **a**   Exclusion is significant as the government is the largest purchaser and provider of services in the country (Hunt and Kirk 2020, 293–294).

308. **c**   A clinical denial is issued when the insurance provider questions a clinical aspect of the admission, such as the LOS of the admission, the level of service, if the encounter meets medical necessity parameters, the site of the service, or if clinical validation is not passed (Casto and White 2021, 219).

309. **a**   CIAs may last for many years and are imposed when serious misconduct (fraud and abuse) is discovered through an audit or self-disclosure. Remediation initiatives, such as training or designation of a compliance officer, are part of the CIA. Remediation activities are intended to offer providers another chance to prove they are worthy of participating in federal healthcare programs (Palkie 2020b, 307).

310. **b**   Though the term valvuloplasty in the index leads to Repair, Replacement, or Supplement, this procedure was performed as a percutaneous Dilation. The root operation Dilation is expanding an orifice or the lumen of a tubular body part (Kuehn and Jorwic 2021).

311. **c**   The False Claims statute also protects whistleblowers. Protections are provided to employees against discharge, demotion, harassment, or discrimination against an employee (Palkie 2020b, 304).

312. **d**   Effective dates of coverage are usually resolved in the front end of the revenue cycle or prior to submission of the bill to payers (Handlon 2020, 264).

313. **b**   When identity theft occurs in the context of medical care, it is known as medical identity theft. Medical identity theft is the inappropriate or unauthorized use of a person's identity to obtain medical goods or services or to falsify claims to fraudulently bill insurance companies (Palkie 2020b, 304).

314. **b**   A low A/R value is favorable (Handlon 2020, 263).

315. **d**   The physician champion, also known in some organizations as the physician advisor, is an individual who assists in communicating with and educating medical staff in areas such as documentation procedures for accurate billing and EHR procedures (Hunt and Kirk 2020, 277).

316. **d**   Preregistration is completed in the front-end process of the revenue cycle. Chargemaster maintenance software and charge capture are utilized in the middle revenue cycle process. Automated claim status and cash posting occur in the back-end processes of the revenue cycle (Handlon 2020, 259).

317. **b**   Since obtaining the patient portion can be a significant challenge for many organizations, permitting electronic payment options through a patient portal is an increasingly popular approach with collections and follow-up (Handlon 2020, 263–264).

318. **b** The correct answer is "N=No" as the condition was not present on admission. The pulmonary embolism developed after admission to the hospital (Hazelwood 2020, 230–231).

319. **b** The concept of a prospective payment system is that charges are calculated before healthcare services are actually provided. The charges are based on historical data on patients with like conditions and procedures. Retrospective payment is payment for the actual cost of services provided (Hazelwood 2020, 225).

320. **c** Patients who are admitted for an HIV-related illness should be assigned a minimum of two codes in the following order: code B20 to identify the HIV disease and additional codes to identify the related diagnosis, which in this case is disseminated candidiasis code B37.7 (Schraffenberger and Palkie 2022, 129).

321. **c** The root operation performed was resection—cutting out or off, without replacement, all of a body part. Even though the entire liver was not removed, the correct root operation is resection based on coding guideline B3.8. PCS contains specific body parts for anatomical subdivisions of a body part, such as lobes of the lungs and liver and regions of the intestine. Resection of the specific body part is coded whenever all of the body part is cut out or off, rather than coding Excision of a less specific body part. The correct code is 0FT20ZZ. The section is Medical and Surgical—character 0; Body System is Hepatobiliary and Pancreas—character F; Root Operation is Resection—character T; Body Part is Liver, Left Lobe—character 2; Approach is Open—character 0; No Device—character Z; and No Qualifier—character Z (Kuehn and Jorwic 2023, 30, 46, 79).

322. **b** Sepsis is a serious medical condition caused by the body's immune response to an infection. Code A41.01 is for sepsis with methicillin-susceptible *Staphylococcus aureus*. Because abdominal pain is a symptom of diverticulitis, only the diverticulitis of the colon is coded (Schraffenberger and Palkie 2022, 43–44, 119–120).

323. **d** The ICD-10-CM index entry for Diabetes, type 1, with gangrene provides E10.52 as the correct code, so the peripheral angiopathy is presumed when gangrene is present (Schraffenberger and Palkie 2022, 43–44).

324. **a** Registering a patient with more than one medical record number is an issue that affects the revenue cycle. Although excess wait time is frustrating for patients, it is not a guarantee of an issue with the revenue cycle. Ensuring the patient's guarantor and employer and completing insurance verification would help the revenue cycle process (Handlon 2020, 249).

325. **a** Local managed contracts, official coding guidelines, and notice of privacy practices are documents in which NCDs and LCDs requirements and revisions are not found. Medicare billing manuals would include these items (Handlon 2020, 247–248).

326. **a** The repair of the hernia is not coded because it was not performed; however, code 0WJG0ZZ is assigned to describe the extent of the procedure, inspection of the peritoneal cavity based on ICD-10-PCS Guideline B3.3. The Z53.09 is also used to indicate the cancelled procedure due to the contraindication. The code R00.1 is also added for the bradycardia that the patient developed during the procedure (Kuehn and Jorwic 2023, 43; Schraffenberger and Palkie 2022, 701).

327. **b** Begin with the main term: Biopsy, artery, temporal (Huey 2021, 24).

328. **a** Assessing the patient's ability to pay for services is the primary responsibility of a financial counselor; the other listed processes are typically performed by a registration staff member (Handlon 2020, 248–249).

329. **d**   Many organizations create policies to follow reasonable registration procedures and occur after medical screening (Handlon 2020, 246).

330. **a**   Present on admission is defined as present at the time the order for inpatient admission occurs—conditions that develop during an outpatient encounter, including emergency department, observation, or outpatient surgery, are considered present on admission. This patient was not admitted with a catheter-associated urinary infection, so that condition cannot be coded as present on admission (POA). The patient was admitted with symptoms of a stroke and diagnoses of COPD and hypertension. The CVA was documented after admission, but the symptoms of the stroke were POA, so this condition would be coded as POA (Hazelwood 2020, 230).

331. **a**   Code 54401 is correct because the prosthesis is self-contained (Huey 2021, 24).

332. **d**   Begin with the main term Relocation; skin pocket; pacemaker (Huey 2021, 24).

333. **c**   Resolving failed edits is one of many duties of the health information management (HIM) department. Various medical departments depend on the coding expertise of HIM professionals to avoid incorrect coding and potential compliance issues (Schraffenberger and Kuehn 2011, 237–238).

334. **c**   One of the responsibilities of the contract management team is to analyze whether discount rates are providing financial incentives that steer the patient population (Handlon 2020, 267).

335. **d**   Edits are used to review a coded claim for accuracy and send back a flag if an error has been detected in the claim. Most organizations run all their claims through edits prior to sending out to any payer to look for errors, correct them, and then send out a clean claim. In this instance the facility has determined to write-off the failed charges because an ABN notice was not signed by the patients (Schraffenberger and Kuehn 2011, 465).

336. **c**   Each Resource-Based Relative Value Scale (RBRVS) comprises three elements: physician work, physician practice expense, and malpractice, each of which is a national average available in the *Federal Register* (Casto and White 2021, 122-123).

337. **a**   A query is routine communication and education tool used to advocate for complete and compliant documentation. The intent is to clarify what has been recorded, not to call into question the provider's clinical judgment or medical expertise. This is an example of a circumstance where the chronic condition must be verified. All secondary conditions must match the definition in the UHDDS and whether the COPD does is not clear (Hunt and Kirk 2020, 285–287).

338. **c**   Utilization management may begin prior to the patient's elective or prescheduled admission or occur after the patient is discharged. Utilization management can be incorporated into all stages of the revenue cycle process through prospective, concurrent, and retrospective reviews. However, most often, utilization management does support the middle-process, but does not ONLY begin after patient admission. Utilization management provides supervision of resources to ensure appropriate utilization of those resources focusing on improving quality and reducing costs. Utilization management incorporates criteria to determine readiness for discharge (Handlon 2020, 252).

339. **a**   Nonparticipating providers (nonPARs) do not sign a participation agreement with Medicare but may or may not accept assignment. If the nonPAR physician elects to accept assignment, he or she is paid 95 percent (5 percent less than participating physicians) of the Medicare fee schedule (MFS). For example, if the MFS amount is $200, the PAR provider receives $160 (80 percent of $200), but the nonPAR provider receives only $152 (95 percent of $160). In this case the physician is nonparticipating so he or she will receive 95 percent of the 80 percent of the MFS or 80 percent of 300, which is $240; 95 percent of the $240 is $228 (Casto and White 2021, 125).

340. **c**   Procedures performed within an orifice on structures that are visible without the aid of any instrumentation are coded to the approach External in the ICD-10-PCS coding system (Kuehn and Jorwic 2023, 54).

341. **d**   HINNs may not be issued to a patient *after* a service is rendered (Handlon 2020, 248).

342. **a**   Remittance advice (RA) files are sent to the provider from the payer with final individual claim adjudication and payment information. RAs provide explanation through itemized claims processing decision information about any adjustments made regarding payment, adjustments, etc. (Handlon 2020, 265).

343. **a**   The policy information provided states this is a single policy or employee-only policy, so the member's spouse is not covered (Casto and White 2021, 16-17).

344. **b**   The insured is the organization that has purchased the insurance policy. In this case, STATE has purchased the insurance coverage for subscriber Jane B. White (Casto and White 2021, 16-17).

345. **c**   Transparency approach involves providing financial information in a user-friendly format along with all relevant past and current patient obligations (Handlon 2020, 267).

346. **d**   A CDI program provides a mechanism for the coding staff to communicate with the physician regarding nonspecific diagnostic statements or when additional diagnoses are suspected but not clearly stated in the record, which helps to avoid assumption coding (Hess 2015, 42).

347. **a**   The hospital-issued notice of noncoverage (HINN) may be provided to patients when an inpatient service has been deemed non-covered due to medical necessity (Handlon 2020, 248).

348. **a**   When coders "optimize" the coding process, they attempt to make coding for reimbursement as accurate as possible. In this way, the healthcare facility can obtain the highest dollar amount justified within the terms of the government program or the insurance policy involved (Hunt and Kirk 2020, 296).

349. **a**   Medical identity theft can be the result of either internal or external forces. Electronic health records have improved the ability to share information, but this has also increased exposure to data making it more vulnerable. Internal medical identity theft is committed by organization insiders, such as clinical or administrative staff with access to patient information. External threats are causing a greater risk for healthcare organizations due to increased threats of ransomware, malware, and denial-of-service (DOS) attacks (Olenik and Reynolds 2017, 290).

350. **a**   The conversion factor is an across-the-board multiplier that sets the allowance for the relative values—a constant (Casto and White 2021, 123).

351. b Utilization management staff work with payers and convey the decision of denial of payment information from commercial payers to patients and families (Handlon 2020, 252).

352. d If a service is hard-coded into the charge description master (CDM), it is important that this decision is communicated to the coding staff. If the decision is not effectively communicated, the result could be duplicate billing that in turn could result in overpayment to the facility (Casto and White 2021, 145).

353. d The ABN's primary purpose is to inform the patient of financial responsibility for outpatient services when it is not likely Medicare will cover due to NCD or LCD requirements (Handlon 2020, 248).

354. c Under the home health prospective payment system (HHPPS), CMS has accounted for nonroutine medical supplies, home health aide visits, medical social services, and nursing and therapy services (Hazelwood 2020, 237).

355. d Unbundling occurs when individual components of a complete procedure or service are billed separately instead of using a combination code (Bowman 2017, 440).

356. c Because clinical documentation improvement (CDI) involves the medical and clinical staffs, it is more likely that the CDI project will be successful if these staff are included in developing the process for documentation improvement. Because all hospital staff do not document in the health record, a memorandum from the CEO to all staff would not be efficient or necessarily effective. The chairperson of the CDI project does not have line authority for employee evaluation. The Joint Commission performs oversight activities but would not be involved in direct operational tasks such as this (Schraffenberger and Kuehn 2011, 360).

357. d All other functions are that of a case manager. Financial counselors are staff dedicated to helping patients and physicians determine sources of reimbursement for healthcare services (Handlon 2020, 248–249).

358. c When an organization has delivered goods or services, payment for the same is expected. Because the revenue has been accrued upon delivery or provision of the goods and services, the organization must have some way to keep track of what is owed to them as a result. Accounts receivable then is merely a list of the amounts due from various customers (in this case, patients). Payment on the individual amounts is expected within a specified period. A schedule of those expected amounts is prepared in order to track and follow up on payments that are overdue (late) (Revoir 2020, 812).

359. a Although historically his cases came out to the moderate level of care average, the physician is ignoring accurate coding rules as well as payer mix. The physician's reimbursement might be middling on average, but that does not mean every payer's reimbursements to him came out that way. Further, his intentional miscoding is inherently fraud. Based on this rationale, all of the other answers are incorrect. Answer d is incorrect because there is intention, which makes the physician's actions fraud (Davis and Doyle 2016, 62–64).

360. c Reviewing and auditing through internal audits enables healthcare facilities to ensure accurate coding and compliance. In this situation, the coding errors made by the lead coder need to be identified and discussed with the lead coder (Casto and White 2021, 208).

361. **a** To meet the CMS's definition of an IRF, facilities must have an inpatient population in which at least 75 percent of the patients require intensive rehabilitation services and one of the following conditions: stroke, spinal cord injury, congenital deformity, amputation, major multiple trauma, fracture of femur, brain injury, neurological disorders, burns, rheumatoid arthritis, systemic vasculitides, osteo-arthritis, polyarthritis, or knee or hip replacement (Hazelwood 2020, 238).

362. **c** Even if the patient is possibly confused or trying to get out of paying the bill, it is in the best interests of the patient and the organization to take her concern seriously and take appropriate measures. This is a potential instance of medical identity theft and the security and compliance departments should be notified so that they can investigate this claim (Davis and Doyle 2016, 82–83).

363. **a** Healthcare entities should consider a policy in which queries may be appropriate when documentation in the patient record fails to meet one of the following five criteria: legibility, completeness, clarity, consistency, and precision (Hunt and Kirk 2020, 285–287).

364. **a** Preauthorization is a term that describes the requirement for a healthcare provider to obtain permission from the health insurer in order to provide predefined services to the patient (Handlon 2020, 247).

365. **d** Under the Medicare hospital outpatient prospective payment system (OPPS), outpatient services such as recovery room, supplies (other than pass-through), and anesthesia are included in this reimbursement method (Casto and White 2021, 107).

366. **a** The patient's first 20 days of care are paid at 100 percent. Days 21–30 are paid all but $170.50 per day; the patient's responsibility is $1,705.00 (10 days x $170.50 per day) (Hazelwood 2020, 213).

367. **a** The Red Flags Rule requires many businesses and organizations to implement a written identity theft prevention program designed to detect the "red flags" of identity theft in day-to-day operations, take steps to prevent the crime, and mitigate its damage (Palkie 2020b, 304–305).

368. **d** The risk of loss in a capitation arrangement rests with the provider. This includes specialists, for example, who provide services upon referral. Without an appropriate referral, the specialist will not be reimbursed. The payer's financial obligation is, for the most part, discharged with the period fixed payments to the provider. On the provider's side, the fixed payments provide a predictable revenue stream. However, because the revenue is not entirely linked to services, the provider is at risk if an unpredicted percentage of the panel (the patients assigned to that provider) uses the provider's services at a high rate (Davis and Doyle 2016, 57).

369. **a** Facilities may design a clinical documentation improvement (CDI) program based on several different models. Improvement work can be done with retrospective record review and queries, with concurrent record review and queries, or with concurrent coding. Although much of the CDI process is often done while the patient is in-house, it does not eliminate the need for post-discharge queries (Schraffenberger and Kuehn 2011, 363).

370. **d** A component of the revenue cycle is claims reconciliation. The healthcare facility uses the explanation of benefits (EOB), Medicare summary notice (MSN), and remittance advice (RA) to reconcile accounts. EOBs and MSNs identify the amount owed by the patient to the facility. Collections can contact the patient to collect outstanding deductibles and copayments. RAs indicate rejected or denied items or claims. Facilities can review the RAs and determine where the claim error can be corrected and resubmitted for additional payment (Casto and White 2021, 173).

371. **c** Educating physicians regarding documentation issues that affect coding is the function of the CDI team. Therefore, that is the best answer (Davis and Doyle 2016, 108).

372. **d** The primary operational components of the CDI program are the record review and the query process. The review process and the physician query process allow for the highest level of quality in clinical documentation (Hess 2015, 158).

373. **b** The purpose of the recovery audit contractors (RAC) program is to reduce improper Medicare payments and prevent future improper payments made of claims of healthcare services to Medicare beneficiaries. Improper payments may be overpayments or underpayments (Rinehart-Thompson 2017e, 258).

374. **a** If the review is a violation of the look-back period clause, all of the other answers are irrelevant (Davis and Doyle 2016, 159).

375. **c** The charge description master can provide a method for grouping items that are frequently reported together. Items that must be reported separately but are used together, such as interventional radiology imaging and injection procedures, are called exploding charges (Schraffenberger and Kuehn 2011, 227).

376. **c** There is a difference between identity theft and medical identity theft and the impact it has on patients. This includes financial and safety concerns regarding care (that is, medical record documentation) (Palkie 2020b, 304).

377. **a** Patient access staff are responsible for entering this data; therefore, it is with that department that HIM needs to work (Davis and Doyle 2016, 4).

378. **d** The Federal Trade Commission has oversight responsibility for identity theft regulations and requires financial institutions and creditors to develop and implement written identity theft prevention programs (Biederman and Dolezel 2017, 406).

379. **b** The purpose of a financial counselor is to assist the patient in understanding their financial obligations and working out a method of payment. This would be the first step (Davis and Doyle 2016, 96–97).

380. **b** When identity theft occurs in the context of medical care, it is known as medical identity theft. Medical identity theft is the inappropriate or unauthorized use of a person's identity to obtain medical goods or services or to falsify claims to fraudulently bill insurance companies (Palkie 2020b, 304).

381. **d** The correct answer is "W=Clinically Undetermined". The physician is unable to clinically determine whether the sepsis was present on admission or not (Hazelwood 2020, 230–231).

382. **c** Answer c is the only option that provides a consistent and reliable method to improve communication and documentation. Options a and b do not provide any communication avenues that will improve documentation or provide coders with necessary information to assign accurate codes. Option d is not appropriate in any case because coders should not be making clinical judgments (Hunt and Kirk 2020, 289).

383. **b** The HIM department can plan focused reviews based on specific problem areas after the initial baseline review has been completed. This would be called a focused inpatient review or focused audit (Schraffenberger and Kuehn 2011, 314–315).

384. **b** The coder assigned the correct diagnosis code. The coder did not assign the correct procedure because the root operation for this procedure is reposition, not supplement. Reposition is moving to its normal location or other suitable location all or a portion of a body part, whereas supplement is defined as putting in or on biological or synthetic material that physically reinforces or augments the function of the portion of a body part (Kuehn and Jorwic 2023, 106-107).

385. **c** Alerts or notification from a consumer reporting agency, suspicious documents, suspicious personally identifying information, patient's reporting, are examples of identity red flag categories (Palkie 2020b, 304).

386. **d** Facilities may design a clinical documentation improvement (CDI) program based on several different models. Improvement work can be done with retrospective record review and queries, with concurrent record review and queries, or with concurrent coding. Although much of the CDI process is often done while the patient is in-house, it does not eliminate the need for post-discharge queries (Schraffenberger and Kuehn 2011, 314–315).

387. **b** Ongoing evaluation is critical to successful coding and billing for third-party payer reimbursement. The goal of internal auditing is to protect providers from sanctions or fines (Palkie 2020b, 308).

388. **c** The length of multiple laceration repairs located in the same classification are added together and one code is assigned (Huey 2021, 82-83).

389. **c** In 2007, Identity Theft Red Flags and Address Discrepancy Rules were enacted as part of the Federal Fair and Accurate Credit Transactions Act (FATCA) of 2003. The FATCA requires financial institutions and creditors to develop and implement written identity theft programs that identify, detect, and respond to red flags that may signal the presence of identity theft (Olenik and Reynolds 2017, 291).

390. **b** As a result of the disparity in documentation practices by providers, querying has become a common communication and educational method to advocate proper documentation practices. Queries can be made in situations when there is clinical evidence for a higher degree of specificity or severity. In this situation the reason for the mechanical ventilation and intubation, most likely, is respiratory failure and the physician would need to be queried for validation of that diagnosis in order for it to be coded (Hunt and Kirk 2020, 285–287).

391. **b** Automated reviews by recovery audit contractors (RACs) allow them to deny payments without ever reviewing a health record. For example, duplicate billing, such as billing for two colonoscopies on the same day for the same Medicare beneficiary, is easy to identify as a potential improper payment. Underpayment and overpayment amounts can be subject to an automated review (Casto and White 2021, 206).

392. **d** A person who reports discriminatory acts or other illegal activity is called a whistleblower. A whistleblower is protected by both a specific federal statute, the Whistleblower Protection Act of 1989, and provisions within individual legislation (Kelly and Greenstone 2020, 111).

393. **c** Episode-of-care payment is a single payment for all care delivered within a defined period of time. This may be an inpatient hospitalization or perhaps outpatient surgery (Hazelwood 2020, 226).

394. **b** 760211 is the charge code which is a unique identifier to specify the service or supply. The number is only meaningful to the organization and does not appear on the billing claim form (Handlon 2020, 256).

395. **c** Each year, the HHS OIG publishes the projects that are planned and the areas identified for review. These published workplans cover CMS and the Administrations for Children and Families and Administration on Aging. The workplan can be found on the HHS OIG website (Hunt and Kirk 2020, 296).

396. **b** When coding lower gastrointestinal endoscopies, coders must distinguish among the following: Proctosigmoidoscopy, which is an examination of the rectum and sigmoid colon; Sigmoidoscopy, which is an examination of the entire rectum, sigmoid colon, and may include part of the descending colon; Colonoscopy, which is an examination of the entire colon, from rectum to cecum, with possible examination of the terminal ileum (Huey 2021, 145).

397. **b** The highest APC receives full payment and the remaining are paid at 50 percent (Hazelwood 2020, 234).

398. **d** The root operation extirpation is defined as taking or cutting out solid material from a body part. The matter may have been broken into pieces during the lithotripsy previous to this encounter, but at this time the pieces of the calculus are being removed (Kuehn and Jorwic 2021).

399. **b** As part of the compliance plan the organization should define what key clinical documents are required based on the care setting and type of record (Hunt and Kirk 2020, 297).

400. **a** Metrics and statistics are about decision making, metrics are important for knowing what is working, how well it is working, and what is not working (Hunt and Kirk 2020, 284).

401. **c** The RBRVS system uses geographic practice code indices to adjust for geography. The conversion factor is a national amount and the practice and malpractice RVUs are not based on geography Hazelwood 2020, 232-233).

402. **b** The answer is "N=No" as the mediastinitis developed following the surgery (Handlon 2020, 230–231).

Domain 5 *Management and Leadership*

403. **a** The use of a recorded webinar is an example of asynchronous learning. Asynchronous learning occurs when the instructor and students are not present at the same time (Kelly and Greenstone 2020, 212).

404. **c** Risks that must be considered for both outsourcing and offshoring include poor security, hidden costs, lack of or improper communication, poor resource management, unbalanced work distribution or dissemination, lack of technology, quality problems, high turnover rates, and legal problems (Kelly and Greenstone 2020, 159).

405. **d** Training is essential to the successful implementation of each new system. The implementation team must define who needs to be trained, who should do the training, how much training is required, and how the training will be accomplished (Biedermann and Dolezel 2017, 260).

406. **c**   A mentor provides advice on developing skills and career options. In this situation Joan is mentoring Sandy towards her goal of becoming a privacy officer (Patena 2020, 732).

407. **c**   The formulary is composed of medications used for commonly occurring conditions or diagnoses treated in the healthcare organization. Organizations accredited by the Joint Commission are required to maintain a formulary and document that they review at least annually for a medication's continued safety and efficacy (Shaw and Carter 2019, 221).

408. **c**   Conflict management focuses on working with the individuals involved to find a mutually acceptable solution. There are three ways to address conflict: compromise, control, and constructive confrontation (LeBlanc 2020, 713).

409. **c**   Individual orientation covers those job duties and responsibilities unique to the person's job in the department (Kelly and Greenstone 2020, 204–205).

410. **c**   Serial work division is the consecutive handling of tasks or products by individuals who perform a specific function in sequence. Often referred to as a production line work division, serial work division tends to create task specialists (Oachs 2020, 764).

411. **a**   To help all members understand the process, a team will undertake development of a flowchart. This work allows the team to thoroughly understand every step in the process and the sequence of steps. It provides a picture of each decision point and each event that must be completed. It readily points out places where there is redundancy and complex and problematic areas (Oachs 2020, 786).

412. **c**   Strategic management is a process a leader uses for assessing a changing environment to create a vision of the future, determining how the organization fits into the anticipated environment based on its mission, vision, and knowledge of its strengths, weaknesses, opportunities, and threats, and then setting in motion a plan of action to position the organization accordingly (McClernon 2020, 916).

413. **b**   Variances are often calculated on the monthly budget report. The organization's policies and procedures manual defines unacceptable variances or variances that must be explained. In identifying variances, it is important to recognize whether the variance is favorable or unfavorable and whether it is temporary or permanent (Revoir 2020, 834).

414. **b**   There must be at least two clinical measures and two human resources indicators for each patient population, defined by internal performance improvement activities. At a minimum, the organization identifies no fewer than two inpatient care areas for which staffing effectiveness data are collected. Identified performance measures relate to processes appropriate to the care and services provided and to problem-prone areas experienced in the past (for example, infection rates or incidences of patient falls). The rationale for indicator selection is based on relevance and sensitivity to each patient area where staffing is planned (Shaw and Carter 2019, 273).

415. **d**   The strategic planning process requires the involvement of each department setting its vision in alignment with the organization and should include the department stakeholders and not be limited by organizational constraints (McClernon 2020, 938–939).

416. **b** The capital budget looks at long-term investments. Such investments are usually related to improvements in the facility infrastructure, expansion of services, or replacement of existing assets. Capital investments focus on either the appropriateness of an investment (given the facility's investment guidelines) or choosing among different opportunities to invest. The capital budget is the facility's plan for allocating resources over and above the operating budget (Revoir 2020, 836).

417. **d** Kinesthetic learners favor a hands-on approach to learning so they can feel and manipulate the material. This may involve clicking through computer screens rather than reading an instruction manual (Kelly and Greenstone 2020, 209).

418. **b** A credential is a formal agreement to practice granted by a professional organization, whereas a license is a legal authorization to practice granted by a by a state (Kelly and Greenstone 2020, 210).

419. **c** After a complaint by a resident, family member, or employees, a Department of Health surveyor may visit a facility at any time to perform a special investigation. This investigation is to ensure that proper is being received by the resident in question and another other within the organization (Shaw and Carter 2019, 342).

420. **a** Organizations that embrace ongoing performance improvement do so because their leaders foster a culture of competence through staff self-development and lifelong learning. The competitive advantage for healthcare organizations today lies in their intellectual capital and organizational effectiveness (Shaw and Carter 2019, 273).

421. **c** After the team develops the preliminary report, surveyors, members of the organization's leadership team, and a representative from the state's licensing agency, if applicable, reconvene for an exit conference. During the exit conference, surveyors summarize their findings and explain any deficiencies identified during the site visit. Leaders have a short opportunity to discuss the surveyors' perspectives or to provide additional information related to any deficiencies (Shaw and Carter 2019, 339).

422. **a** Deemed status means accrediting bodies such as the Joint Commission can survey facilities for compliance with the Medicare Conditions of Participation for hospitals instead of government (Rinehart-Thompson 2017e, 253).

423. **a** A contract action arises when one party claims that the other party has failed to meet an obligation set forth in a valid contract. Another way to state this is that the other party has breached the contract. The resolution available is either compensation or performance of the obligation (Rinehart-Thompson 2020, 54).

424. **c** In-service education is a continuous process that builds on the basic skills learned through new employee orientation and on-the-job training. It is concerned with teaching employees specific skills and behaviors required to maintain job performance (Patena 2020, 733).

425. **c** There are several laws that affect discrimination in employment on the basis of race, color, religion, age, sex, national origin, citizenship status, and veterans status. Most organizations would like to hire someone whose vision for the organization is in line with their own vision (Reynolds and Brodnik 2017c, 490).

426. **c** Consumer engagement activities both educate the consumer and make them more responsible for their personal health and health information. Patient portal training helps the consumer to better manage their own health information (Kelly and Greenstone 2020, 208–209).

427. **d**   Alternative staffing structures offer flexibility in hours, location, and job responsibilities as a method to attract and retain employees and eliminate staffing shortages. Some examples are job sharing, outsourcing, flextime, and telecommuting (Oachs 2020, 768).

428. **b**   The Americans with Disabilities Act of 1990 protects individuals with disabilities. Employees must be able to perform the necessary functions of a job with "reasonable accommodations," which include modifications to the workplace or conditions of employment so that a disabled worker can perform the job (Reynolds and Brodnik 2017c, 492).

429. **a**   Innovation should.be seen as an essential part of strategic thinking rather than a replacement or additional part of management (McClernon 2020, 919).

430. **d**   Zero-based budgets apply to organizations for which each budget cycle poses the opportunity to continue or discontinue services based on the availability of resources. Every department or activity must be justified and prioritized annually in order to effectively allocate the organization's resources. Professional associations and charitable foundations, for example, routinely use zero-based budgeting (Revoir 2020, 831).

431. **b**   Regardless of the counseling and disciplinary actions mandated by the organization, managers should take some key steps of their own such as documenting the steps taken to improve performance (LeBlanc 2020, 712).

432. **d**   The opening conference, a meeting conducted at the beginning of the accreditation site visit during which the surveyors outline the schedule of activities and list any individuals whom they would like to interview, is an important opportunity for the organization to set the tone for the survey process (Shaw and Carter 2019, 335).

433. **b**   The key to implementation or achieving its strategies is identifying goals to achieve each strategy. Visioning and forecasting are key to identifying strategies not implementation (McClernon 2020, 933).

434. **d**   Licensure is a state's act of granting a healthcare organization or an individual healthcare practitioner permission to provide services of a defined scope in a limited geographical area. State governments issue licenses based on regulations specific to healthcare practices (Shaw and Carter 2019, 330).

435. **a**   An aspect of infection surveillance involves employee health and illness tracking. Employees are a critical vector for bringing community-acquired infections into healthcare settings. Policies related to the tracking of employee absences exist for the specific purpose of preventing infection via healthcare workers. Reports of employee absences are tabulated and examined for any possible connection to cases of HAI (Shaw and Carter 2019, 181).

436. **d**   Strategic management is a process a leader uses for assessing a changing environment to create a vision of the future, determining how the organization fits into the anticipated environment based on its mission, vision, and knowledge of its strengths, weaknesses, opportunities, and threats, and then setting in motion a plan of action to position the organization accordingly (McClernon 2020, 916).

437. **b**   Each provider who practices care under the auspices of a healthcare organization must do so in accordance with delineated clinical privileges. One of the requirements for these privileges is for the individual to carry his or her own professional liability insurance and therefore that provider is considered an independent contractor within the healthcare organization (Shaw and Carter 2019, 279).

438. **a** The implementation plan outlines each strategy and then details how to achieve the strategy using goals and objectives (McClernon 2020, 933–934).

439. **c** Internal candidates are individuals that are already employed by an organization. One of the advantages of hiring an internal candidate is that the candidate is a proven employee with an understanding of the organization. Hiring internal candidates can also improves the morale and a sense of loyalty for current employees (Kelly and Greenstone 2020, 157).

440. **a** Recruitment is the process of finding, soliciting, and attracting new employees. However, the manager should be sure to understand the organization's recruitment and hiring policies and to seek the assistance of the HR department before the vacancy is publicized (LeBlanc 2020, 701).

441. **c** Strategic managers develop skills reflecting the implications and opportunities afforded by trends. Whether reading a journal or discussing new ideas with others, strategic managers are always testing new ideas, identifying those that have merit, and discarding those that do not. They are creating links between the trends and the value-adding actions they can take (McClernon 2020, 918).

442. **c** The second part of the CARF accreditation is the document review. The document review is an in-depth study in which accreditation surveyors examine an organization's policies and procedures, administrative rules and regulations, administrative records, human resources records, and the case records of patients (Shaw and Carter 2019, 341).

443. **b** Like any organization, the medical staff, as a self-governing entity, needs to have structure. The medical staff bylaws provide an organizational structure to ensure communication with the governing body and high-quality patient care. Committees are used to help most medical staffs function. This committee structure is used to make credentialing and clinical privilege decisions (Reynolds and Brodnik 2017b, 476–478).

444. **b** The needs analysis is critical to the design of the training plan. This approach typically focuses on three levels: the organization, the specific job tasks, and the individual employee (Patena 2020, 722).

445. **b** All contracts include representations or warranties of some sort, which are statements of facts existing at the time the contract is made. These statements are made by one party to induce the other party to enter the contract. Typically, these statements relate to the quality of goods or services purchased or leased (Klaver 2017b, 129–130).

446. **a** Blended learning uses several delivery methods thereby gaining the advantages and reducing the disadvantages of each method alone (Patena 2020, 743).

447. **b** Agreements between the covered entity and a business associate include: requiring the business associate to make available all of its books and records relating to protected health information (PHI) use and disclosure to the Department of Health and Human Services or its agent; prohibiting the business associate from using or disclosing PHI in any way that would violate the HIPAA Privacy Rule; and prohibiting the business associate from using or disclosing PHI for any purpose other than that described in the contract with the covered entity; and other agreements. But it does not allow the business associate to maintain PHI indefinitely (Rinehart-Thompson 2017c, 211–212).

448. **b** A strategy map is a tool that provides a visual representation of an organization's critical objectives and the relationships among them that drive organizational performance. Depicting change as a road map is a useful way to help others understand the goals and the course of change (McClernon 2020, 941).

449. **b** Job analysis data is collected to determine job requirements and delineate appropriate position classification and grade-level assignments (Kelly and Greenstone 2020, 136).

450. **c** The accreditation committee performs mock surveys and identifies gaps between actual performance and optimal performance relative to accreditation standards (Kelley and Greenstone 2020, 225–226).

451. **c** All healthcare organizations are mandated by regulation to examine care processes that have a potential for error that can cause injury to patients. NPSG 01.01.01 states that two patient identifiers are used when administering medications, blood, or blood components (Shaw and Carter 2019, 163–164).

452. **c** Getting employees opinion is part of the internal assessment. The other options are external groups (McClernon 2020, 921–923).

453. **c** In cross-training, the employee learns to perform the jobs of many team members. This method is most useful when work teams are involved (Patena 2020, 732).

454. **d** Flextime generally refers to the employee's ability to work by varying his or her starting and stopping hours around a core of midshift hours, such as 10 a.m. to 1 p.m. Depending on their position and the institution, employees may have a certain degree of freedom in determining their hours (Oachs 2020, 767).

455. **a** The strategic profile identifies the existing key services or products of the department or organization, the nature of its customers and users, the nature of its market segments, and the nature of its geographic markets (McClernon 2020, 922; Robert 2006, 53–542).

456. **a** The purpose of hold harmless or indemnification clauses is to either transfer or assume liability. For example, the indemnitor (party assuming liability) may agree to hold the other party harmless against claims arising from the indemnitor's own actions or failures to act. This means if actions (or inactions) result in harm to the other party, the indemnitor will seek to make that party whole, often through some sort of compensation (Klaver 2017b, 129–130).

457. **d** The needs analysis is the first step to the design of a training and development plan. This approach typically focuses on three levels: the organization, the specific job tasks and the individual employee (Patena 2020, 722).

458. **a** Appointments to the board of directors is important information, but the Joint Commission requires detailed information on the responsibilities and actions of the board, not necessarily its composition. The Joint Commission requires healthcare organizations to collect data on each of these areas: medication management, blood and blood product use, restraint and seclusion use, behavior management and treatment, operative and other invasive procedures, and resuscitation and its outcomes (Shaw and Carter 2019, 304, 313).

459. **d** Sometimes problems arise because of conflicts among employees. It is common for people to disagree, and sometimes a difference of opinion can increase creativity. However, too much conflict can also waste time, reduce productivity, and decrease morale. When taken to the extreme, it can threaten the safety of employees and cause damage to property (LeBlanc 2020, 713).

460. **d** The rapidly changing landscape in healthcare requires the strategic planning process be open to change to achieve the vision and strategy (McClernon 2020, 920).

461. **b** The items, other than answer b, are operational improvements, and involving consumers is innovative and a breakthrough strategy (McClernon 2020, 917).

462. **b** Healthcare organizations need to be very clear about which abbreviations are not acceptable to use when writing or communicating medication orders. The organization's policy should also define whether or when the diagnosis, condition, or indication for use is included on a medication order (Shaw and Carter 2019, 222–223).

463. **b** SWOT analysis looks at the internal strengths of an organization or department, and the external opportunities and threats. These are considered to be elements that the department can control. In this scenario there is a weakness due to the outdated chart tracking software that is not compatible with the digital dictation system (Kelly and Greenstone 2020, 30–31).

464. **b** Once the budget preparation period is over and budget reports are issued, the budget becomes a controlling tool. The other examples occur when the budget is being used as a planning tool (Kelly and Greenstone 2020, 72).

465. **b** Alternate work schedules are alternatives to the regular 40-hour workweek; the following are examples: compressed workweek, flextime, and job sharing (Oachs 2020, 767).

466. **c** The payback period is the time required to recoup the cost of an investment. Mortgage refinancing analysis frequently uses the concept of payback period. Mortgage refinancing is considered when interest rates have dropped. Refinancing may require up-front interest payments and called points as well as a variety of administrative costs. In this example, the payback period is the time it takes for the savings in interest to equal the cost of the refinancing (Revoir 2020, 839).

467. **c** To be legally enforceable under civil law, a contract must comply with any applicable state and federal laws, and it must meet the following conditions: it must describe an agreement between two or more person or entities, it must include a valid offer, acceptance of the offer, and consideration (Klaver 2017b, 127–128).

468. **c** Human resources needs to provide training to managers on how to calculate performance appraisal results in relation to pay-for-performance ratings (Kelly and Greenstone 2020, 188).

469. **c** The strategic goals and objectives need to be clearly outlined, with assignments for who will be accountable, timelines, allocation of resources, and measurements that will be used to ensure success of implementation. When a detailed implementation includes the elements laid out clearly—with timeframes and regular updates provided within the organization—the likelihood of strategic success increases significantly (McClernon 2020, 934).

470. **c**   A process measure has a scientific basis for it. In this example, the percentage of antibiotics administered before surgery has been proven through evidence-based medicine, so it is scientifically based (Shaw and Carter 2019, 40–41).

471. **b**   It is unfavorable and permanent because money that was not in the budget was spent on consulting services (Revoir 2020, 834).

472. **c**   When the operating budget has been developed and approved, it is the responsibility of the department manager to ensure the budget goals are met and to explain all variances (Revoir 2020, 833).

473. **a**   Empowerment is the concept of providing employees with the tools and resources to solve problems themselves. Employees obtain power over their work situation by assuming responsibility (Patena 2020, 750).

474. **a**   Effective change management leadership influences rapid, profound and sustainable behavior change (Amatayakul 2019, 160).

475. **b**   When a manager is planning to contract for staffing in a transitional situation in order to meet organizational goals, various types of contracts can be considered. In this situation, a full service contract would be used. Contracting for staff to handle a complete function (ROI in this case) within the department is a full service contract (Oachs 2020, 769).

476. **b**   Monitoring and controlling are distinct processes, but in project management they work together as a single activity. The monitoring activity is performed to determine the current status of the project, enabling the project to be controlled. The control activity is performed to assess project status in reference to planned activities and their timeline. If he project is off target, a project manager would take action to bring it back on track (Shaw and Carter 2019, 371).

477. **d**   Encouraging team productivity can be a major issue in many organizations. This is an outgrowth of the two common management styles used by most organizations. One style is inclusive: all viewpoints are considered with respect to their potential contribution to solving the PI issue at hand. The other style is exclusive: its goal is to get to a result as quickly as possible. Each style has positive and negative aspects (Shaw and Carter 2019, 60).

478. **b**   Organizing is the way in which an organization or work unit is designed and operated to attain desired goals; it involves how tasks are grouped and ensures resources are allocated appropriately (Swenson 2020, 655).

479. **c**   The mission statement sets the core purpose of an organization or group (Swenson 2020, 654).

480. **d**   The spaghetti diagram (also called a movement diagram) is a visual depiction of the layout of workspace with movements of people and items superimposed on top; this tool is used to evaluate workflow (Oachs 2020, 785).

481. **c**   The early majority adopter group comprise the backbone of the organization, are conventional and deliberate in their decisions, and for a bridge with other adopter categories (Swenson 2020, 673).

482. **b**   Flexibility refers to the fact that controls must be adaptable to real changes in the requirements of a process (Oachs 2020, 776).

483. **d**   It is important to take time for new employee training; feedback will provide information from employees as to whether they are comfortable with their new job after the orientation (Patena 2020, 725–729).

484. **a**   The ADA requires employers to provide reasonable accommodations for physical or mental limitations with regard to many employment-related functions, including training (Patena 2020, 756).

485. **d**   Brooks's Law states that adding people to a team actually slows down team productivity due to adjustment to different work styles, learning curve, low team cohesion, and time for task orientation (Swenson 2020, 671–672).

486. **c**   Layoffs are similar to terminations except that they are essentially unpaid leaves of absence initiated by employer as a strategy for downsizing staff in response to a change in the organization's status (LeBlanc 2020, 713).

487. **c**   Employees have the right to disagree with management and can express their opinions or complaints in a variety of ways. Organizations establish grievance procedures that define the steps an employee can follow to seek resolution of a disagreement they have with a management on a job-related issue (LeBlanc 2020, 7144).

488. **d**   The collection of accounts comprising assets, liabilities, owner's equity, revenues and expenses comprise the general ledger (Revior 2020, 820).

489. **c**   Scope, budget, and schedule are the project constraints and directly relate to how the project is planned (Olson 2020, 852).

490. **b**   Lewin identified three stages of change that are the basis for many change management approaches used today. In the "refreezing" step, interventions ensure that there is no way back to the old processes (Amatayakul 2017, 172).

491. **c**   In the context of work performance, when variations are identified, further analysis is needed (Oachs 2020, 777).

492. **d**   The systems model includes input, process, output, controls and standards, feedback, and the external environment. The external environment includes factors beyond the organization control such as regulations, accreditation requirements, and the labor market (Oachs 2020, 782). ffl

493. **d**   The laggard adopter group serve a purpose of keeping the organization from changing too fast (Swenson 2020, 673).

494. **d**   A job (position) description outlines the work to be performed by a specific employee or group of employees with the same responsibilities (LeBlanc 2020, 699).

495. **b**   The journal entry to record a cash payment transaction is to debit cash and credit accounts receivable (Revior 2020, 819-820).

496. **a**   The project charter defines the project and the corresponding constraints (Olson 2020, 868).

497. **c** The goal of benchmarking is to improve performance by measuring and comparing a selected work process, identifying best practices, and perhaps conducting interviews with the benchmark organization or organizations. Opportunities for process improvement can be identified where best practice has been applied in other organizations. A benchmark organization is usually an organization of similar size and other characteristics. Before embarking on a benchmarking project, coding managers should determine the criteria or indicators for the benchmark comparison (Shaw and Carter 2019, 42).

498. **a** In this instance, Jane is a leader. A leader is an individual who ahs commanding authority or influence (Kelly and Greenstone 2020, 2).

499. **d** Revenue is the recognition of income earned and the use of appropriated capital from the rendering of services during the current period. In this example, radiology procedures would be a form a revenue for the outpatient imaging center (Kelly and Greenstone 2020, 72).

500. **c** A job specification is a document (or a section of the job description document) that is focused on the knowledge, skills, abilities, and characteristics required of an individual in order to perform the job (LeBlanc 2020, 700).

501. **c** Punitive damages may also be awarded to the employee as a way to further punish the employer and prevent the employer's discriminatory behavior from continuing (Kelly and Greenstone 2020, 111).

502. **c** Of the four major components or stages of strategic planning, the only answer is monitoring the external environment as it is part of the Environmental assessment. Budget's come after the strategic plan and a consultant is optional as is setting up committees (McClernon 2020, 920).

503. **b** Job crafting is the redefinition of a job by an individual to incorporate his or her own motives, strengths, and passions. It is the action that employees take to shape, mold, and redefine their jobs (Kelly and Greenstone 2020, 147).

504. **a** The commonly used point method determines a specific wage or salary (LeBlanc 2020, 709).

505. **d** General guidelines include holding a private meeting in which you explain your position, are quick and concise, are firm with the decision, are prepared with termination information and paperwork, and treat the person respectfully (LeBlanc 2020, 712–713).

506. **c** Knowledge management applies to the learning environment in an organization as well as the transfer of knowledge and skills from one generation of workers to the next (Kelly and Greenstone 2020, 52).

507. **c** After factoring in the two changes, the final budget target was $120,000 with a target schedule of 19 months (Olson, 876–878).

508. **a** A 360-degree interview involves three different interviews, with the supervisor of the position, peers of the position, and subordinates of the position (Kelly and Greenstone 2020, 164).

509. **a** The diffusion theory states that how quickly an innovation is adopted depends on a number of factors such as if there is an advantage, how easy it is to understand, and the degree results are visible to others (Swenson, 2020, 675)

510. **d** Reasonable accommodation means the adjustment cannot place an undue hardship on the employer. The concept of an undue hardship will vary among employers (Kelly and Greenstone 2020, 108-109).

511. **c** Legitimate authority identifies individuals who have the right to demonstrate power over other individuals within a bureaucratic organization (Kelly and Greenstone 2020, 4).

512. **d** The income statement summarizes the organization's revenue and expense transactions during the fiscal year. The income statement can be prepared at any point in time and reflects results up to that point. The income statement contains only revenue and expense accounts and reflects only the activity for the current fiscal year (Revior 2020, 820).

513. **c** The job specification section of the job description is where a manager can list the requirements of the position including professional certifications (LeBlanc 2020, 700).

514. **c** With a telecommuting option, employees work full- or part-time in their own homes. The EHR has enabled more employees to work remotely (Oachs 2020, 768).

515. **a** The concurrent handling of tasks is called parallel work division. Multiple employees do the same tasks from beginning to end (Oachs 2020, 764).

516. **a** A vision statement describes the ideal and desired future state toward which an organization strives (Swenson 2020, 654).

517. **a** Kurt Lewin's change theory suggests that refreezing, or making the change status quo, is necessary as the last step of the change process (Swenson 2020, 679).

518. **c** The 85/15 rule states that 85 percent of issues are related to systems and processes and only 15 percent are related to unproductive employees. Daniel should observe the process first (Swenson 2020, 651).

519. **b** Personal motivation is the most powerful way for someone to change. Personal motivation needs to be stimulated when there is an external factor causing the change (Amatayakul 2017, 161).

520. **b** The Gantt chart is used for project management to show how components of a task are scheduled over time (Swenson 2020, 648).

Practice Exam 1 Answers

Domain 1 *Data and Information Governance*

1. **c** Laws and regulations determine how long records must be retained by the facility. The facility must then set aside money and physical space or server space for all of those records to meet those laws and regulations (Reynolds and Morey 2020, 135–136).

2. **a** The chief complaint or reason for the visit is the nature and duration of the symptoms that caused the patient's illness and caused the patient to seek medical attention as stated in the patient's own words. In this scenario the patient came in complaining of abdominal pain, so this is the chief complaint (Reynolds and Morey 2020, 109).

3. **b** Data quality needs to be consistent. A difference in the birth dates provides a good example of how the lack of consistency can lead to problems (Sharp and Madlock-Brown 2020, 202).

4. **d** A discharge summary must be completed within 30 days after discharge for most patients but within 24 hours for patients transferred to other facilities. Discharge summaries are not always required for patients who were hospitalized for less than 48 hours (Reynolds and Morey 2020, 116–117).

5. **d** Authentication means to prove authorship and can be done in several ways. Methods of electronically signing documentation include a digital signature (a digitized image of a signature), a biometric identifier such as fingerprint or retinal scan, or a code or password. The physician assistant and charge nurse cannot authenticate the physician's entry in lieu of the physician as it is the physician's documentation. Likewise, having the HIM clerk use a physician's signature stamp is not an accepted method of authentication (Reynolds and Morey 2020, 126–127).

6. **b** Charting by exception is a method of documenting only abnormal or unusual findings or deviations from the prescribed plan of the care. A complete patient assessment is performed every shift. When events differ from the assessment or the expected norm for a particular patient, the notes should focus on that particular event and include the data, assessment, intervention, and response. The purpose of charting by exception is to reduce repetitive recordkeeping and documentation of normal events (Reynolds and Morey 2020, 114).

7. **a** Resident assessment protocols (RAPs) form a critical link to decisions about care planning and provide guidance on how to synthesize assessment information within a comprehensive assessment. The triggers target conditions for additional assessment and review, as warranted by Minimum Data Set (MDS) item responses. The RAPs guidelines help facility staff evaluate triggered conditions (James 2017b, 328).

8. **b** A review of the identified duplicates and overlays often reveals procedural problems that contribute to the creation of errors. Although health information management (HIM) departments may be the hub of identifying, mitigating, and correcting master patient index (MPI) errors, that information may never be shared with the registration department. Registration process improvement activities can eventually reduce work for HIM departments (Reynolds and Morey 2020, 133).

9. **c** Record reviews that are conducted while a patient is still in the facility are considered concurrent reviews (Reynolds and Morey 2020, 125).

10. **d**   A data set is defined as a list of recommended data elements with uniform definitions that are relevant for a particular use. Data sets are used to encourage uniform data collection and reporting (Johns 2015, 277).

11. **d**   Structured data commonly refer to data that are organized and easy to retrieve and to interpret by traditional databases and data models. The data elements in a patient's automated laboratory order, or result, are coded and alphanumeric. Their fields are predefined and limited. In other words, the type of data is discrete, and the format of this data is structured (Johns 2020, 83).

12. **b**   The content of the emergency health record should generally include the time and means of arrival, treatment rendered, and instructions at discharge. Facilities are required to do a pertinent history, including the chief complaint and onset of illness or injury but not a complete medical history of the patient (Reynolds and Morey 2020, 118–119).

13. **a**   An indicator is a performance measure that enables healthcare organizations to monitor a process to determine whether it is meeting process requirements. Monitoring blood sugars on admission and discharge is an indicator of the quality of care delivered to the diabetes patient during the stay (Shaw and Carter 2019, 143).

14. **b**   Metadata are often referred to as "data about data." Metadata are structured information used to increase the effective use of data. One of the most familiar types of metadata is used to describe data in databases. Data element name, data type, and field length are examples of this kind of metadata (Johns 2020, 83).

15. **b**   The Minimum Data Set (MDS) is a component of the resident assessment instrument (RAI) and is used to collect information about the resident's risk factors and to plan the ongoing care and treatment of the resident in the long-term care facility (James 2017b, 325–326).

16. **c**   Ownership of the health record is generally granted to the healthcare provider who generates the record. Since the record serves as both a medical document and as a legal document that provides proof of care, it is the business record of the healthcare provider (Fahrenholz 2017a, 45).

17. **b**   Facilities should maintain all information related to patient diagnosis and treatment methods in the patient record. Only information related to appointment timeframes and insurance and billing correspondence should not be made part of the record (Reynolds and Morey 2020, 118).

18. **d**   A source-oriented format is when information is categorized according to its supplier or source (in the case of a hospital, this could be by department) (Reynolds and Morey 2020, 121).

19. **a**   The HIM professional should do comparative performance data. Comparative performance data, such as nursing home compare in this case, allows facilities to determine how the facility does in comparison to similar facilities. Facilities report their performance and in turn, the facilities have access to data from these measures. The comparison can assure the organization that it is performing up to industry standards or help the organization identify opportunities for improvement (Shaw and Carter 2019, 356–357).

20. **c**   Except in emergency situations, every surgical patient's chart must include a report of a complete history and physical before the surgery is to be performed (Reynolds and Morey 2020, 110).

21. **c** This type of data would be found on a dashboard report provided to the hospital's board of directors. The measures show a dramatic change in patient safety issues at this organization. The increase in each measure result supports a decline in overall quality of care. The board would now need to investigate to determine why these changes occurred (Shaw and Carter 2019, 322–323).

22. **a** As the HIM department merges two duplicate records together, the source system (laboratory) also must be corrected. This creates new challenges for organizations because merge functionality could be different in each system or module, which in turn creates data redundancy. Addressing ongoing errors within the MPI means an established quality measurement and maintenance program is crucial to the future of healthcare (Glondys and Kadlec 2017, 488).

23. **b** Authorship is the origin of recorded information that is attributed to a specific individual or entity. Electronic tools make it easier to copy and paste documentation from one record to another or to pull information forward from a previous visit, someone else's records, or other sources either intentionally or inadvertently. The ability to copy and paste entries leads to a record where a clinician may, upon signing the documentation, unwittingly swear to the accuracy and comprehensiveness of substantial amounts of duplicated, inapplicable, misleading, or erroneous information (Amatayakul 2017, 505).

24. **c** The documentation that comprises the legal health record (LHR) may physically exist in separate and multiple paper-based or electronic systems. This complicates the process of pulling the entire legal record together in response to authorized requests to produce the complete patient record. Once the LHR is defined, it is best practice to create a health record matrix that identifies and tracks the physical location of each paper document and the source of each electronic document that constitutes the LHR. In addition to defining the content of the LHR, it is best practice to establish a policy statement on the maintenance of it (Rinehart-Thompson 2020, 58).

25. **d** The clinical documentation that is entered into the patient record as text is not as easily automated due to the unstructured nature of the information. Unstructured clinical information includes notes written by physicians and other practitioners who treat the patient, dictated and transcribed reports, and legal forms such as consents and advance directives (Biedermann and Dolezel 2017, 84).

26. **b** The American Health Information Management Association (AHIMA) recommends that records be destroyed in such a way that the information cannot possibly be reconstructed. The destruction should be documented, and the documentation should include the following: date of destruction, method of destruction (shredding, burning, or other means), description of the disposed record series of numbers or items, inclusive dates covered, a statement that the records were destroyed in the normal course of business, and the signatures of the individuals supervising and witnessing the destruction. AHIMA further recommends that facilities maintain destruction certification documents permanently. Such certificates may be required as evidence that records were destroyed in the regular course of business. When facilities fail to apply destruction policies uniformly or when destruction is contrary to policy, courts may allow a jury to infer that the facility destroyed its records to hide evidence (Reynolds and Morey 2020, 140).

27. **c** Data governance is an emerging practice in the healthcare industry. Decision-making and authority over data-related matters is data governance. It is clear that any industry as reliant on data as healthcare needs a plan for managing this asset (Biedermann and Dolezel 2017, 163).

Domain 2 *Compliance with Access, Use, and Disclosure of Health Information*

28. **a**   In order to maintain patient privacy, certain audits may need to be completed daily. If a high-profile patient is currently in a facility, for example, access logs may need to be checked daily to determine whether all access to this patient's information by the workforce is appropriate (Thomason 2013, 173).

29. **d**   The Privacy Rule establishes a patient's right to receive an accounting of disclosures of their PHI made by a covered entity (Brinda and Watters 2020, 325).

30. **a**   The documentation that comprises the legal health record (LHR) may physically exist in separate and multiple paper-based or electronic systems. This complicates the process of pulling the entire legal record together in response to authorized requests to produce the complete patient record. Once the LHR is defined, it is best practice to create a health record matrix that identifies and tracks the physical location of each paper document and the source of each electronic document that constitutes the LHR. In addition to defining the content of the LHR, it is best practice to establish a policy statement on the maintenance of it (Rinehart-Thompson 2020, 57–58).

31. **a**   All states have a health department with a division that is required to track and record communicable diseases. When a patient is diagnosed with one of the diseases from the health department's communicable disease list, the healthcare provider must notify the public health department. Measles is a condition that should be reported within 24 hours to the health department (Shaw and Carter 2019, 177).

32. **c**   Unless specifically protected by law (generally a statute), incident reports tend to be discoverable. This is particularly true if the incident report is disseminated or its presence is made known in a discoverable document (Rinehart-Thompson 2020, 68–69).

33. **c**   The process of disclosing health record documentation originally created by a different provider is called redisclosure. In the interest of patient care, health records from other facilities should be made part of the designated record set at the current facility if that information is needed for diagnosis or treatment, and if state law does not otherwise prohibit it (Rinehart-Thompson 2017c, 231–232).

34. **d**   Audit logs are a chronological set of computerized records that provides evidence of a computer system utilization (log-ins and log-outs, file accesses) used to determine security violations (Brinda and Watters 2020, 334–335).

35. **a**   This situation must be corrected. The privacy officer should complete a process flow and identify the areas where a breakdown in the process is resulting in a complaint of mailing the report to the wrong patient. It is important for the covered entity to take as many precautions as possible to ensure compliance by its workforce. Training is necessary in this situation to mitigate this type of error (Rinehart-Thompson 2017d, 255–256).

36. **c**   Virtual private network (VPN) uses a secure tunnel through a public network, usually the Internet, to connect remote sites or users. Security procedures include firewalls, encryption, and server authentication (Amatayakul 2017, 335).

37. **b**   Role-based access control (RBAC) is a control system in which access decisions are based on the roles of individual users as part of an organization (Theodos 2017, 270).

38. **a** Before an organization can decide on the methods for conducting the security risk analysis, they must consider their own characteristics and environment and implement reasonable and appropriate measures to protect against reasonably anticipated threats and hazards to the security of PHI. The security risk analysis process provides covered entities and business associates with the structural framework upon which to build their security plan (Biedermann and Dolezel 2017, 381).

39. **c** The privacy rule requires a covered entity to arrange a convenient time and place for the individual to inspect his or her record. However, the covered entity also has an obligation to protect the record's integrity. Therefore, it is within the covered entity's right to provide an authorized HIM staff member to be present when the individual reviews the record (Rinehart-Thompson 2017d, 245–246).

40. **c** Competent adults have a general right to consent to or refuse medical treatment. If an adult has a sound mind or did when he or she created a living will, this patient has the right to refuse treatment (Klaver 2017c, 154–155).

41. **c** Treatment, payment, and healthcare operations (45 CFR 164.501)—collectively referred to as TPO—are functions of a covered entity (CE) that are necessary for the CE to successfully conduct business. It is not the intent of the Privacy Rule to impose onerous rules that hinder a CE's functions. Therefore, many of the Privacy Rule's requirements are relaxed or removed where PHI is needed for purposes of TPO (Rinehart-Thompson 2017c, 216).

42. **c** A facility may maintain a facility directory of patients being treated. HIPAA's Privacy Rule permits the facility to maintain in its directory the following information about an individual if the individual has not objected: name, location in the facility, and condition described in general terms. This information may be disclosed to persons who ask for the individual by name (Rinehart-Thompson 2017c, 227).

43. **b** If the data breach impacts 500 or more individuals, the covered entity or business associate must notify the secretary of the Department of Health and Human Services (HHS) within 60 days of date of discovery of the breach. If the number of individuals impacted by the breach exceeds 500, a healthcare organization must notify and report the incident to the local media (Brinda and Watters 2020, 320).

44. **c** The custodian of health records is the individual who has been designated as having responsibility for the care, custody, control, and proper safekeeping and disclosure of health records for such persons or institutions that prepare and maintain records of healthcare (Brodnik 2017a, 9).

45. **c** Generally, if the patient is a minor at the time of treatment or hospitalization but has reached the age of majority at the time the authorization for access or disclosure of information is signed, the patient's authorization is legally required (Brodnik 2017b, 343–344).

46. **c** The HIPAA Privacy Rule provides patients with significant rights that allow them to have some measure of control over their health information. As long as state laws or regulations or the physician does not state otherwise, competent adult patients have the right to access their health record (Rinehart-Thompson 2017c, 224–225).

47. **c** The signature of the attending physician, next of kin, and insurance are not necessary on a HIPAA Complaint Authorization form. The notice of privacy practices informs a patient how and when PHI can be released. If a particular use of information is not covered in the notice of privacy practices, the patient must sign an authorization form specific to the additional disclosure before his or her information can be released (Brinda and Watters 2020, 324).

48. **b** Covered entities (CEs) must respond to requests to access PHI within 30 days. There can be a further 30-day extension however, but the first response must be within 30 days (Rinehart-Thompson 2017d, 245).

49. **b** Those who choose to destroy the original health record may do so within weeks, months, or years of scanning. If the record was destroyed according to guidelines for destruction and no scanned record exists, the certificate of destruction should be presented in lieu of the record (Reynolds and Morey 2020, 139–140).

50. **a** The Privacy Rule provides patients an opportunity to agree or object to specific types of disclosure. These do not require a written authorization; verbal authorization is acceptable. However, communication with the patient regarding these types of disclosures and the patient's decision should be documented in the health record or other appropriate manner of documentation (Brinda and Watters 2020, 327).

51. **c** Hospitals strive to keep incident reports confidential, and in some states, incident reports are protected under statutes protecting quality improvement studies and activities. Incident reports themselves should not be considered a part of the health record. Because the staff member mentioned in the record that an incident report was completed, it will likely be discoverable as the health record is already a discoverable document (Rinehart-Thompson 2020, 68–69).

Domain 3 *Data Analytics and Informatics*

52. **d** Telehealth is the use of electronic information and telecommunications technologies to support long-distance clinical healthcare, patient and professional health-related education, public health, and health administration (Lee-Eichenwald 2020, 370).

53. **d** The HIE's record locator service (RLS) manages the pointers to the information on the servers of the HIE participants. The pointers in a RLS can include a person identification number (person ID) and metadata. The RLS does not provide information about the record, it merely points to where it might be found. Data are not stored in a centralized database and records are only provided when queried (Lee-Eichenwald 2020, 388–389).

54. **d** The unique identifier in the patient table is the patient number. It is unique to each patient. Patient last name, first name, and date of birth can be shared with other patients, but the identifier will not (Biedermann and Dolezel 2017, 189).

55. **b** A many-to-many relationship occurs only in a data model developed at the conceptual level. In this case, the relationship between patients and consulting physicians is many-to-many. For each instance of patient, there could be many instances of consulting physician because patients can be seen by more than one consulting physician. For each instance of consulting physician, there could be many patients because the physician sees many patients (Sayles and Kavanaugh-Burke 2021, 47-48).

56. **b** Most organizations recognize that commercial products can meet their needs and that most of these products will far surpass the functionality that could be self-developed. Still, some organizations want to at least consider the build option. Some physicians are intrigued with developing their own perfect system, and some hospitals have development teams they do not want to give up. An organization's decision to build or buy should be based on a careful review of the marketplace. Currently, it is more expensive to undertake self-development. Unless self-development is coupled with a vendor partnership that leads to commercialization, a self-developed system can be a drawback when attempting to integrate with commercial products as the organization grows, merges, or acquires affiliates (Amatayakul 2017, 191).

57. **c** A table is an orderly arrangement of values that groups data into rows and columns. It should have specific, understandable headings for every column and row (White 2020a, 198).

58. **c** The gross death rate is the proportion of all hospital discharges that ended in death. It is the basic indicator of mortality in a healthcare facility. The gross death rate is calculated by dividing the total number of deaths occurring in a given time period by the total number of discharges, including deaths, for the same time period: $25/500 = 0.05 \times 100 = 5\%$ (Edgerton 2020, 487).

59. **c** Running a mock query would be part of application testing that ensures every function of the new computer system works. Application testing also ensures the system meets the functional requirements and other required specifications in the RFP or contract (Sayles and Kavanaugh-Burke 2021, 100).

60. **b** Normalization is a formal process applied to database design to determine which variables should be grouped in a table to reduce data redundancy. In this example, entering the patient's last name and first name into separate fields is normalization (Johns 2015, 132).

61. **a** The disease index is a listing in diagnosis code number order for patients discharged from the facility during a particular period (Sharp and Madlock-Brown 2020, 178).

62. **b** The work distribution chart should be completed by the employee and it includes all responsible task content as well as hours spent on tasks over a designated period of time (Oachs 2020, 766).

63. **b** In data mining, the analyst performs exploratory data analysis to determine trends and identify patterns in the data set. Data mining is sometimes referred to as knowledge discovery. In healthcare, data mining may be used to determine if it is cost effective to expand facilities (White 2020b, 520).

64. **b** A pie chart is an easily understood chart in which the sizes of the slices of the pie show the proportional contribution of each part. Pie charts can be used to show the component parts of a single group or variable. In this case, the intent is to show the proportion of each payer to the whole payer mix (Marc 2020, 537).

65. **c** The incidence rate is a computation that compares the number of new cases of a specific disease for a given time period to the population at risk for the disease during the same time period (Edgerton 2020, 494).

66. **c** Data conversion refers to the fact that data is already automated in one system but needs to be put into another, most often new, system—which is not always an easy task depending on the nature of the software and application programming language used. Chart conversion or transition refer to converting data on paper to electronic form and data processing refers to processing any data in a computer (Amatayakul 2020, 427).

67. **d**   The patient meets the severity of illness with the vaginal bleeding but does not meet intensity of service because the surgery is not being performed as an inpatient. She would not meet the admission criteria provided (Shaw and Carter 2019, 143).

68. **d**   Boolean search capabilities such as "and," "or," and "not" may be used in the QBE database to narrow down the data to specifically what the user needs. In this example the query could retrieve patients who had a diagnosis cerebral infarction or cerebral hemorrhage and find all of them (Sayles and Kavanaugh-Burke 2021, 40).

69. **b**   Monitoring results enables a hospital to understand if the present system is currently supporting the needs of the organization and whether the next step, identify needs, will set in motion new or further development or acquisition of health IT (Amatayakul 2020, 434).

70. **b**   The average length of stay (ALOS) is calculated from the total LOS. The total LOS divided by the number of patients discharged is the ALOS. Using the data provided, the ALOS for the 9 patients discharged on April 1 is 6 days (54/9) (Edgerton 2020, 485).

71. **b**   Project plans are key to correctly implementing new systems because a key part of their functionality is to identify dependencies among tasks (Amatayakul 2020, 417).

72. **a**   The opt-in model requires patients to specifically affirm their desire to have their data made available for exchange within an HIE. This option provides up-front control for patients since their data cannot be included unless they have agreed (Biedermann and Dolezel 2017, 306).

73. **c**   The weight of each MS-DRG is multiplied by the number of discharges for that MS-DRG to arrive at the total weight for each MS-DRG. The total weights are summed and divided by the number of total discharges to arrive at the case-mix index for a hospital. Calculation is as follows: $(0.8642 \times 10) + (0.6521 \times 20) + (1.2987 \times 10) + (0.8402 \times 20) + (0.6418 \times 10) = 57.893/70 = 0.8270$ (White 2021, 164).

74. **a**   Super users are individuals with normal jobs who happen to be skilled at learning new information technology and can help others master new technology; they are not intended to replace scribes, trainers, or technicians (Amatayakul 2020, 421).

75. **d**   The HIE's record locator service (RLS) manages the pointers to the information on the servers of the HIE participants. The pointers in a RLS can include a person identification number (person ID) and metadata. The RLS does not provide information about the record, it merely points to where it might be found. Data are not stored in a centralized database and records are only provided when queried (Lee-Eichenwald 2020, 388–389).

76. **b**   Because of the number of tasks and their complexity and dependencies in EHR implementation, it is important to have an issues management program. An issues management program serves to receive and document issues and track them to their resolution (Amatayakul 2017, 258).

77. **b**   Data provenance refers to the ability to track the source of data; the other choices are functions that describe or help maintain data (Amatayakul 2020, 407).

78. **b**   A Pareto chart is a kind of bar graph that uses data to determine priorities in problem solving. The Pareto principle states that 80 percent of costs or problems are caused by 20 percent of the patients or staff (Shaw and Carter 2019, 85–86).

79. **b** It is often not feasible to adopt all components from a single vendor, but even when it is, interoperability with other providers is not assured. Only adoption of standards provides the greatest (though not absolute) interoperability. An application service provider does not address interoperability across vendors. A systems view is very helpful, but does not afford the same level of assurance that application of cross-industry standards provides (Amatayakul 2020, 412, 415, 439).

80. **b** The primary key (PK) for PATIENT, PATIENT_MRN, is repeated in VISIT, as is the PK for CLINIC, CLINIC_ID. These keys are called foreign keys (FK) in the VISIT table. Foreign keys allow relationships between tables. By having the foreign keys in VISIT, the information in PATIENT and CLINIC is linked through the VISIT table (Johns 2015, 128–129).

81. **b** Monitoring results enables a hospital to understand if the present system is currently supporting the needs of the organization and whether the next step, identify needs, will set in motion new or further development or acquisition of health IT (Amatayakul 2020, 434).

82. **a** Source systems are not just clinical systems, but also include administrative and financial systems. The technology includes patient monitoring equipment, dispensing devices and robotics, and supporting infrastructure of networks, cloud-based storage, and telehealth technologies (Sayles and Kavanaugh-Burke 2021, 199).

83. **c** The use of health information technology, including EHRs, can help to prevent errors that occur in the delivery of care. This leads to improved outcomes and patient care (Sayles and Kavanaugh-Burke 2021, 198, 201).

84. **b** Reminders can notify physicians of screenings that should be performed based on the patient's age and gender. In this example, the physician could receive a reminder that the patient is due for an MMR immunization (Sayles and Kavanaugh-Burke 2021, 201).

85. **b** The primary key (PK) for PATIENT, PATIENT_MRN, is repeated in VISIT, as is the PK for CLINIC, CLINIC_ID. These keys are called foreign keys (FK) in the VISIT table. Foreign keys allow relationships between tables. By having the foreign keys in VISIT, the information in PATIENT and CLINIC is linked through the VISIT table (Johns 2015, 127–128).

Domain 4 *Revenue Cycle Management*

86. **a** The anemia D50.0 was not specified as acute and would be sequenced first based on principal diagnosis guidelines followed by the code N93.8 for the dysfunctional uterine bleeding (Schraffenberger and Palkie 2022, 94, 179).

87. **c** Haldol is a drug frequently administered for behavior or mental conditions, so the coder would suspect mental or behavioral problems for this patient. The physician must be queried to confirm the diagnosis. Documentation is needed in the record to support the coding of the mental or behavioral problem (Hunt and Kirk 2020, 285–286).

88. **b** The root operation performed was division—cutting into a body part without drawing fluids or gases from the body part in order to separate or transect a body part. The intent of the operation was to separate the femur, so 0Q860ZZ is the correct code. The Section is Medical and Surgical—character 0; Body System is Lower Bones—character Q; Root Operation is Division—character 8; Body Part is Upper Femur, Right—character 6; Approach is Open—character 0; No Device—character Z; and No Qualifier—character Z (Kuehn and Jorwic 2023, 30, 101-102).

89. **c** Medical identity theft occurs when a patient uses another person's name and insurance information to receive healthcare benefits. Most often this is done so a person can receive medical care with an insurance benefit and pay less or nothing for the care he or she receives (Rinehart-Thompson 2020, 67).

90. **b** The patient was admitted for diabetic cataract. There is a causal relationship given between the diabetes and the cataract, so E11.36 would be assigned. This follows the UHDDS guidelines for principal diagnosis selection. The correct root operation is replacement because the intraocular lens was inserted at the time of the cataract extraction. Replacement is putting in or on biological or synthetic material that physically takes the place or function of all or a portion of a body part (Schraffenberger and Palkie 2022, 94, 196-198; Kuehn and Jorwic 2023, 30, 129-130).

91. **d** Upcoding describes using diagnoses or procedure codes that are selected specifically because they result in higher payment from third-party payers (Hunt and Kirk 2020, 296).

92. **a** Outpatient coding guidelines do not allow coding of possible conditions as a diagnosis for the patient. Do not code diagnoses documented as "probable," "suspected," "questionable," "rule out," "working diagnosis," or other similar terms indicating uncertainty. Rather, code the condition(s) to the highest degree of certainty for that encounter or visit, such as symptoms, signs, abnormal test results, or other reasons for the visit (Schraffenberger and Palkie 2022, 105).

93. **a** Clustering is the practice of coding or charging one or two middle levels of service codes exclusively under the philosophy that, although some will be higher and some lower, the charges will average out over an extended period (Huey 2021, 408).

94. **d** The cause of every transfusion reaction, the signs, symptoms, or conditions suffered by a patient as the result of the administration of an incompatible transfusion, must be investigated. Most deaths resulting from hemolytic transfusion reactions were primarily attributable to incomplete patient identification processes for blood verification (Shaw and Carter 2019, 162).

95. **b** The increased awareness of duplication of services increased the drive to determine the medical necessity for treatments and care. Purchasers and payers of healthcare services began to demand a more comprehensive approach to care—one that decreased costs and improved the quality of care provided. Along with this demand came standards intended to ensure that the services provided were timely, cost-efficient, and appropriate to the patient's medical condition. As patients were stuck with medical bills that insurance companies refused to pay and providers were unwilling to write off because they were not deemed medically necessary, new processes were developed to address these concerns (Shaw and Carter 2019, 134).

96. **b** Capitated rate is a method of payment for health services in which the third-party payer reimburses providers a fixed, per capita amount for a period. *Per capita* means per head or per person. A common phrase in capitated contracts is per member per month (PMPM). The PMPM is the amount of money paid each month for each individual enrolled in the health insurance plan. Capitation is characteristic of HMOs (Casto and White 2021, 55).

97. **a** HIM professionals should be involved in the development and management of the chargemaster. These codes and charges must be updated at least annually (Sayles and Kavanaugh 2021, 149).

98. **d** Electronic data interchange (EDI) allows the transfer (incoming and outgoing) of information directly from one computer to another by using flexible, standard formats. This technology was first used in healthcare for the billing function (Sayles and Kavanaugh-Burke 2021, 282).

99. **c** These procedures have been unbundled. Unbundling is the practice of coding services separately that should be coded together as a package because all the parts are included within one code and, therefore, one price. Unbundling done deliberately to obtain a higher reimbursement is a misrepresentation of services and can be considered fraud (Huey 2021, 409).

100. **d** Workers' compensation is a payer that pays for healthcare services due to work-related incidents. Because workers' compensation is paying the bill, they are the third-party (Casto and White 2021, 46).

101. **c** In addition to improving the coding process, CDI also improves and supports eata quality, availability, and usability—all key aspects of data governance. The quality of this documentation is vital in order to properly evaluate patient care, meet all regulatory requirements, and obtain the appropriate amount of reimbursement (Sayles and Kavanaugh-Burke 2021, 150).

102. **c** A query may not be appropriate because the clinical information or clinical picture does not appear to support the documentation of a condition or procedure. In situations in which the provider's documented diagnosis does not appear to be supported by clinical findings, a healthcare entity's policies can provide guidance on a process for addressing the issue without querying the attending physician (Hunt and Kirk 2020, 285–287).

103. **b** Episode-of-care reimbursement is a healthcare payment method in which providers receive one lump sum for all the services they provide related to a condition or disease. This payment methodology is also referred to as bundled payment methodlogy(Casto and White 2021, 55, 57).

104. **d** The ethical obligations of the health information management (HIM) professional include placing service before self-interest. The HIM professional must ensure the honor of the profession before personal advantage as well as the health and welfare of patients before all other interests (Swirsky 2020, 895).

105. **a** The health information manager must continuously promote complete, accurate, and timely documentation to ensure appropriate coding, billing, and reimbursement. This requires a close working relationship with the medical staff, perhaps through the use of a physician advisor. Physician advisors assist in educating medical staff members on documentation needed for accurate billing. The medical staff is more likely to listen to a peer than to a facility employee, especially when the topic is documentation needed to ensure appropriate reimbursement (Hunt and Kirk 2020, 277).

106. **b** The explanation of benefits (EOB) is a report from a third-party payer that is sent from a healthcare insurer to the policy holder and provider. The EOB describes how the claim was processed by the healthcare insurer. It will include the actual charge for the service, the allowable amount under the payer agreement, the amount paid to the provider, and the remaining balance (if any) that the policy holder is obligated to pay (Casto and White 2021, 172).

107. **d** Recovery audit contractors (RACs) carry out the provisions of the National Recovery Audit Program. RACs work with a mission of reducing Medicare improper payments through detection and collection of overpayments, identification of underpayments, and implementation of actions that will prevent future improper payments (Casto and White 2021, 204).

108. **b** The quality of the documentation entered in the health record by providers can have major impacts on the ability of coding staff to perform their clinical analyses and assign accurate codes. In this situation, the best solution would be to educate the entire medical staff on their roles in the clinical documentation improvement process. Explaining to them the documentation guidelines and what documentation is needed in the record to support the more accurate coding of diabetes and its manifestations will reduce the need for coders to continue to query for this clarification (Hunt and Kirk 2020, 283–284).

109. **c** The closed reduction of the fracture is coded because it is the main procedure. The laceration repair is also coded. A –59 modifier would need to be added to the laceration code to indicate a distinct procedural service for billing purposes. When more than one classification of wound repair is performed, all codes are reported with the code for the most complicated procedure listed first (Huey 2021, 24, 82, 98-99).

110. **c** The "X" qualifier is used for biopsies (diagnostic) that are excision, extraction and drainage procedures (Kuehn and Jorwic 2023, 77).

111. **b** As a result of the disparity in documentation practices by providers, querying has become a common communication and educational method to advocate proper documentation practices. Queries can be made in situations when there is clinical evidence for a higher degree of specificity or severity (Hunt and Kirk 2020, 285–287).

112. **d** Integrated delivery system (IDS) is a term referring to the collaboration integration of healthcare providers. The goal of the IDS is a seamless delivery of care along the continuum of care, so one bill would be generated (Fuller 2020, 26).

113. **d** The error rates are not comparable since there is no data about the number of records coded during the period by each coder. Work measurement is the process of studying the amount of work accomplished and the amount of work it takes to accomplish it. It involves the collection of data relevant to the work (Oachs 2020, 775).

114. **c** A claim scrubber is used by facilities as an internal auditing system to limit the number of denied claims (Casto and White 2021, 167-168).

115. **a** Preauthorization, or prior authorization, occurs when the provider obtains permission to provide the service from the insurance carrier, usually to ensure the patient has the benefits available. Precertification is when the insurance carrier must review the proposed service or procedure and approve it as medically necessary before payment will be granted to the provider (Handlon 2020, 247).

116. **d** As part of the move to pay for value, CMS developed their value-based purchasing (VBP) program as part of the Affordable Care Act. This VBP program includes four domains: safety, clinical care, efficiency and cost reduction, and person and community engagement. Each domain includes a variety of measures that must be reported to CMS regularly. The HCAHPS survey results are part of the Person/Community Engagement domain (Shaw and Carter 2019, 135–136).

117. **c** A term or series of terms that appear in parenthesis following a main term or subterm are known as nonessential modifiers. The presence or absence of these parenthetical terms in the diagnosis statement has no effect on the selection of codes listed for that main term or subterm (Schraffenberger and Palkie 2022, 14).

Domain 5 *Management and Leadership*

118. **b** A standard is performance criteria designed for the purpose of assessing factors such as quality, productivity, and performance (Oachs 2020, 771).

119. **c** A charge of negligent hiring can be made if a current employee commits a serious offense and it can be shown that the organization should have known about the employee's tendencies had a thorough background check been done prior to hiring (Kelly and Greenstone 2020, 162).

120. **c** Many employers pay a slightly higher hourly wage to employees who work less desirable shifts (evening, night, weekend). This is referred to as shift differential (Oachs 2020, 767).

121. **a** Strategic management and thinking should be seen as an essential part of management rather than a replacement or additional part of management. It is an expected part of the role of managers, not just senior leaders (McClernon 2020, 918–919).

122. **a** Performance management is a set of tools and practices for setting performance goals and designing sustainable job improvement strategies with employees, monitoring employee progress toward job performance goals with feedback. New managers should always be trained on the organization's methods for evaluating employee performance (Kelly and Greenstone 2020, 179).

123. **c** The on-site Joint Commission survey utilizes a tracer methodology that permits assessment of operational systems and processes in relation to the actual experiences of selected patients currently under the organization's care. Patients are selected on the basis of the current census of patients that the organization identifies as typical of its case mix. As cases are examined in relation to the actual care processes, the surveyor may identify performance issues or trends in one or more steps of the process or in the interfaces between processes. Patients on subsequent days may be selected on the basis of issues raised (Shaw and Carter 2019, 335).

124. **d** Under the provisions of FLSA, covered groups are referred to as nonexempt employees (LeBlanc 2020, 708).

125. **c** Balanced scorecard methodology is a technique for measuring organization performance across the four perspectives of customer, financial, internal processes, and learning and growth (McClernon 2020, 941).

126. **b**   Based on the content in the scenario, it can be deduced that Jake is reviewing the record of care standards. These standards should be detailed enough so the patient can be identified and should also support the care provided to include diagnosis, treatments, care results, and communication between staff. Care providers should also document patient progress in the patient record. This information is used to make care decisions (Shaw and Carter 2019, 360).

127. **a**   Review of diversity practices and sexual harassment training take place at the organizational level of orientation training (Kelly and Greenstone 2020, 203).

128. **b**   The difference between the budgeted fees and actual fees is an unfavorable variance of $2,000. Unfavorable variances occur when the actual results are worse than what was budgeted (Revoir 2020, 834).

129. **d**   American Health Information Management Association (AHIMA) professionals must abide to the AHIMA Code of Ethics principle to refuse to participate in or conceal unethical practices or procedures (Swirsky 2020, 895).

130. **a**   The agreements that are reached in a participant agreement or vendor contract should be developed into operational policies and procedures (Lee-Eichenwald 2020, 396).

131. **b**   Credentialing is the process of reviewing and validating qualifications, granting professional or medical staff membership, and awarding delineated privileges. Specific policies and procedures are used by healthcare organizations to accomplish this process. The credentialing process verifies the education, training, experience, current competence, and ability to perform the privileges requested as well as any other background information pertinent to an individual requesting medical staff membership (Fahrenholz 2017b, 79–80).

132. **d**   Performance measurement is the process of comparing the outcomes of an organization, work unit, or employee to pre-established performance standards. The results of performance measurement are usually expressed as percentages, rates, ratios, averages, or other quantitative assessment. It is used to assess quality and productivity in clinical and administrative services. An 18 percent error rate on abstracting data is an indicator of a process problem in the health information management (HIM) department because it is an HIM function. The other items are not under the control of the HIM department and would not indicate a process problem in HIM (Oachs 2020, 776).

133. **b**   In reengineering, the entire manner and purpose of a work process is questioned. The goal is to achieve the desired process outcome in the most effective and efficient manner possible. The results expected from reengineering efforts include increased productivity, decreased costs, improved quality, maximized revenue, and more satisfied customers. However, it should be clearly understood that the main focus is on reducing costs (Oachs 2020, 791).

134. **b**   Strategic thinking is a way of introducing innovation into decision-making and engaging others in the process of change. The skills that distinguish a strategic thinker include the ability to plan and strategize, flexibility and creativity, comfort with uncertainty and risk, a sense of urgency and vision of how to move change forward positively, being able to gain a powerful core of organizational supporters and customers, and the capability to communicate the vision and plans (McClernon 2020, 917–918).

135. **a**   Home health agencies are expected to conduct an assessment that accurately reflects the patient's current health status and includes information to establish and monitor a plan of care. The plan of care must be reviewed and updated at least every 60 days or as often as the severity of the patient's condition requires (Selman-Holman 2017, 349).

136. **c** After employees have been recruited and selected, the first step is to introduce them to the organization and their immediate work setting and functions. New employee orientation includes a group of activities that introduce the employee to the organization's mission, policies, rules, and culture; the department or workgroup; and the specific job he or she will be performing (Patena 2020, 725–726).

137. **c** The second step after documenting employee performance issues is to develop an action plan incorporating SMART goals (Kelly and Greenstone 2020, 195).

138. **b** Voluntary turnover occurs when an employee chooses to leave an organization (Kelly and Greenstone 2020, 166).

139. **c** The current ratio compares total current assets with total current liabilities:

$$\frac{4,000,000}{5,000,000} = \frac{4}{5} = 0.8$$

$$\frac{\text{Total current assets}}{\text{Total current liabilities}}$$

From this information, one can take the current assets (cash + accounts receivable + inventory) divided by current liabilities (accounts payable) to arrive at current ratio. The current ratio indicates that for every dollar of current liability, $0.80 of current assets could be used to discharge the liability, which is not enough because it is not at least $1 (Revoir 2020, 823).

140. **d** In this case, a profitability index helps the organization prioritize investment opportunities. For each investment, divide the present value of the cash inflows by the present value of the cash outflows. The profitability index for each investment is calculated in the figure below. Each investment is equally profitable, as all three have the same profitability index of 4 (Revoir 2020, 840–841).

	Radiology	Cardiology	Pharmacy
Present value of cash inflows	$2,000,000	$1,200,000	$40,000
Present value of cash outflows	$500,000	$300,000	$10,000
Profitability Index	$2,000,000/$500,000 = 4	$1,200,000/$300,000 = 4	$40,000/$10,000 = 4

141. **b** Performance standards establish how well and how much work must be accomplished which guides performance expectations (LeBlanc 2020, 700).

142. **d** Voluntary reviews are conducted at the request of the healthcare facility seeking accreditation or certification (Shaw and Carter 2019, 330).

143. **a** SWOT analysis looks at the internal strengths of an organization or department, and the external opportunities and threats. These are considered to be elements that the department can control. In this scenario having the coding staff credentialed and up to date on continuing education is a strength for this department (Kelly and Greenstone 2020, 30–31).

144. **d** Visual learners use the sense of sight to best learn new material. They prefer written instructions and material over being told how to do a task (Kelly and Greenstone 2020, 209).

145. **d** Accreditation approval is based on whether the organization voluntarily meets a set of accreditation standards developed by the accreditation agency that serve as the basis for comparative assessment during the review or survey process and confirm the quality of the services that healthcare organizations provide (Shaw and Carter 2019, 330).

146. **a** When a manager is planning to contract for staffing in a transitional situation in order to meet organizational goals, various types of arrangements can be considered. Full-service contracting would be handing off a complete function to the contracted company (Oachs 2020, 769).

147. **c** Granting clinical privileges refers to the authorizing of a practitioner to provide specific patient care services within well-defined limits. The criteria for awarding clinical privileges must be detailed in the medical staff bylaws or rules and regulations (Fuller 2020, 16).

148. **b** In-service education is a continuous process that builds on the basic skills learned through new employee orientation and on-the-job training. In-service education is concerned with teaching employees specific skills and behaviors required to maintain job performance or to retrain workers whose jobs have changed (Patena 2020, 733).

149. **b** Job shadowing is a method in which one employee follows another employee to observe certain functions of their job. The intent is that the experienced employee educates the new employee on specific aspects of their job (Kelly and Greenstone 2020, 208).

150. **a** People learn best in different ways, such as auditorily and visually. To accommodate these differences, a variety of methods should be used in training (Sayles and Kavanaugh-Burke 2021, 101-102).

Practice Exam 2 Answers

1. **d** If an admission clerk is not careful about reviewing patient accounts with the same name and other identifying elements in the MPI, then a new account for the patient will be created under a new medical record number. The physician will then not have the information from any previous admissions to review and utilize for the current admission (Reynolds and Morey 2020, 132).

2. **c** Health records and other documentation related to patient care are the property of the hospital or healthcare provider that created them. However, the information in each record belongs to the individual patient (Fahrenholz 2017a, 45).

3. **c** Precision often relates to numerical data. It denotes how close to an actual size, weight, or other standard a particular measurement is (Sharp and Madlock-Brown 2020, 202).

4. **b** The employee turnover rate is over the internal benchmark for this hospital, so a performance improvement (PI) team should be formed to determine what the causes for this increase were. This increase in the turnover rate represents an opportunity for improvement (Shaw and Carter 2019, 27–28).

5. **c** The operative report should be written or dictated immediately after surgery and filed in the patient's health record as soon as possible. Some hospitals may require surgeons to include brief descriptions of the operations in their postoperative progress notes when delays in dictation or transcription are unavoidable. Other caregivers can then refer to the progress note until the final operative report becomes available (Reynolds and Morey 2020, 115).

6. **a** A consultation report is the documented findings or recommendation for further treatment by a physician or specialist. Consultations are usually performed at the request of the attending physician (Reynolds and Morey 2020, 113).

7. **b** The Abbreviated Injury Scale reflects that nature of the injury and the severity (threat to life) by body system. It may be assigned manually by the registrar or generated as part of the database from data entered by the trauma registrar (Sharp and Madlock-Brown 2020, 182).

8. **d** The steps in developing a record retention program include: conducting an inventory of the facility's records, determining the format and location of record storage, assigning each record a retention period, and destroying records that are no longer needed (Reynolds and Morey 2020, 137).

9. **d** Data stewards are typically designated throughout the enterprise within business units, including IT (Johns 2020, 93).

10. **d** Researchers use convenience samples when they "conveniently" use any unit that is at hand. For example, HIM professionals investigating physician satisfaction with departmental services could interview physicians who came to the department (White 2020a, 239).

11. **a** The physician principally responsible for the patient's hospital care generally dictates the discharge summary. Regardless of who documents it, the attending physician is responsible for the content and quality of the summary and must date and sign it (Jenkins 2017, 155–156).

12. **d** An updated entry may be used for the patient's history and physical when the patient is readmitted within 30 days of the initial treatment for the same condition (Reynolds and Morey 2020, 110).

13. **c** Data management is based on the assumption that all data have a life cycle. Typical data life cycle functions requiring data governance include: establishing what data are to be collected and how they are to be captured; setting standards for data retention and storage; determining processes for data access and distribution; establishing standards for data archival and destruction (Johns 2020, 82).

14. **c** Sometimes, the organizational characteristic or parameter about which data are being collected occurs too frequently to measure every occurrence. In this case, those collecting the data might want to use sampling techniques. Sampling is the recording of a smaller subset of observations of the characteristic or parameter, making certain, however, that a sufficient number of observations have been made to predict the overall configuration of the data (Shaw and Carter 2019, 72).

15. **b** A pathology report is a document that contains the diagnosis determined by examining cells and tissues under a microscope. The report may also contain information about the size, shape, and appearance of a specimen as it looks to the naked eye (Reynolds and Morey 2020, 115).

16. **d** A vocabulary standard is a common definition for medical terms to encourage consistent descriptions of an individual's condition in the health record (Sayles and Kavanaugh-Burke 2021, 43-44).

17. **b** The results of the inventory indicate a significant problem and should not be ignored. Before in-service training or memos can be developed, the organization's formal position on data dictionaries must be established through development of a policy and associated standards. An organization-wide data dictionary is developed outside the framework of a specific database design process. This data dictionary serves to promote data quality through data consistency across the organization. Individual data element definitions are agreed upon and defined. This leads to better quality data and facilitates the detailed, technical data dictionaries that are integrated with the databases themselves (Sharp and Madlock-Brown 2020, 203).

18. **c** The delivery of healthcare is increasingly complex; therefore, the related workflows are also increasingly complex. As the use of technology becomes critical in all aspects of patient care, understanding how the workflows within and between processes is critical. The success of information technology projects is not solely dependent on the technology, but also on the people and the process. Workflow analysis would uncover the human and process problems and should be done any time work involves multiple departments or functions and prior to identifying an information technology (IT) solution (Oachs 2020, 795).

19. **a** The answer is a because the primary physician and other direct care providers are the only ones that can document diagnosis and treatment information in the record (Reynolds and Morey 2020, 101, 127).

20. **c** Structured data commonly refer to data that are organized and easily retrievable and interpreted by traditional databases and data models (Johns 2020, 83).

21. **a** Although registries and databases are almost universally computerized, data collection is sometimes done manually. The most frequent method is abstracting, the process of reviewing the patient health records and entering the required data elements into the database (Sharp and Madlock-Brown 2020, 197).

22. **a** An accession number consists of the first digits of the year the patient was first seen at the facility, with the remaining digits assigned sequentially throughout the year. The first case in, for example, might be 09-0001. The accession number may be assigned manually or by the automated cancer database used by the organization. An accession registry of all cases can be kept manually or be provided as a report by the database software (Sharp and Madlock-Brown 2020, 180).

23. **a** These data are showing that Doctor X bills code 99213 primarily and not the other four service codes for established patients. However, the graph tells the reader nothing about Doctor X's documentation which would make answers b and c incorrect. Doctor X does use 99212 less than his peers, not more than his peers. A physician who consistently reports the same level of service for all patient encounters may look suspicious to claims auditors. With the exception of certain specialists, physicians treat all types of patients in their offices, and office treatment requires use of most of the levels of services (Huey 2021, 313-314).

24. **a** The destruction of patient-identifiable clinical documentation should be carried in accordance with relevant federal and state regulations as well as organizational policy. Health records related to open investigations, audits, or court cases should not be destroyed for any reason. Paper-based health records can be destroyed using any of the following methods: burning, shredding, pulping, or pulverizing (Fahrenholz 2017b, 107).

25. **c** Reliability is a measure of consistency of data items based on their reproducibility and an estimation of their error of measurement (Sharp and Madlock-Brown 2020, 202).

26. **c** Medicare Conditions of Participation require that admitting physicians perform an initial physical examination within 24 hours of admission. Documentation of medical history, consents, and the physical examination must be available in the patient's record before any surgical procedures can be performed (Reynolds and Morey 2020, 110).

27. **a** The graph shows that the Asian population has increased in the last five years, so the organization may need to adjust staffing, offer a wider variety in dietary choices, and ensure patient rights and safety are appropriate in the face of possible language barriers and cultural differences (Shaw and Carter 2019, 90).

Domain 2 *Compliance with Access, Use, and Disclosure of Health Information*

28. **c** A patient portal would allow the patient to access this information. The ONC has defined a patient portal as a secure online website that gives patients convenient 24-hour access to personal health information from anywhere with an Internet connection (Sandefer 2020, 457).

29. **a** The purpose of a notice of privacy practices is to inform patients of how a healthcare provider may use and share the patient's health information (Brinda and Watters 2020, 318).

30. **b** Emancipated minors generally may authorize the access and disclosure of their own PHI. If the minor is married or previously married, the minor may authorize the disclosure or use of his or her information. If the minor is under the age of 18 and is the parent of a child, the minor may authorize the access and disclosures of his or her own information as well as that of his or her child (Brodnik 2017b, 343–344).

31. **b** Breach notification laws do exist in numerous states, but they often are not tailored to medical information (Rinehart-Thompson 2020, 68).

32. **c** Context-based authentication is the most stringent type of access control. It takes into account the person attempting to access the data, the type of data being accessed, and the context of the transaction in which the access attempt is made (Sayles and Kavanaugh-Burke 2021, 295).

33. **a** The patient portal allows a patient to access all or part of the health record that is maintained by the patient's provider (Amatayakul 2017, 15).

34. **b** Entity authentication is the verification of a user's identity. Simply put, this standard seeks to ensure that organizations put methods in place to verify that users are who they claim they are (Biedermann and Dolezel 2017, 395).

35. **c** A firewall is a computer system or a combination of systems that provide a security barrier or support an access control policy between two networks or between a network and other traffic outside the network. This gatekeeper is physicially located between the routes of a public network like the Internet and those of a private network (Sayles and Kavanaugh-Burke 2021, 299).

36. **b** The security audit process should include triggers that identify the need for a closer inspection. Just because a trigger has been activated does not mean that there has been a breach. With common names such as Smith and Jones, it would be easy for an employee named Smith or Jones to access patient information for an unrelated person with the same last name (Sayles and Kavanaugh-Burke 2021, 298).

37. **b** As within any type of setting, a common security threat to a health information system is an internal threat within the organization by employees (Amatayakul 2017, 371–372).

38. **c** Audit logs are used to facilitate the determination of security violations and to identify areas for improvement. In this case, the audit log review should be used to begin an investigation into what exactly the employee printed and why (Brinda and Watters 2020, 334–335).

39. **d** The distinction of psychotherapy notes is important due to HIPAA requirements that these notes may not be released unless specifically identified in an authorization (Rinehart-Thompson 2017c, 222).

40. **c** The HIPAA Privacy Rule concept of "minimum necessary" does not apply to disclosures made for treatment purposes. However, the covered entity must define, within the organization, what information physicians need as part of their treatment role (Rinehart-Thompson 2017c, 234).

41. **c** The Privacy Rule's general requirement is that authorization must be obtained for uses and disclosure of protected health information (PHI) created for research that includes treatment of the individual (Rinehart-Thompson 2017c, 225).

42. **b** The e-discovery process includes the pretrial activities wherein participants acquire and analyze any electronic data that could be used in civil or criminal legal proceedings. Some of the aspects addressed in e-discovery include the format of the data, the location of the accumulated data, and record retention and destruction protocols (Rinehart-Thompson 2020, 63).

43. **c** Allowing employees of a covered entity to access their own protected health information electronically results in a situation in which the covered entity may be in compliance with parts of the HIPAA Privacy Rule, but in violation of other sections of the Privacy Rule. An ideal situation would be to establish a patient portal through which all patients may view their own records in a secure manner, and for which an employee has neither more or less rights than any other patient (Thomason 2013, 109).

44. **b**   By virtue of their age, minors are generally considered legally incompetent and unable to consent to their own treatment. Therefore, the consent of a parent or other legal guardian is required. If the minor's parents are divorced, only one parent needs to consent for treatment (Klaver 2017c, 160).

45. **a**   This question requires a differentiation among different types of documentation that may exist in the health record. Option a is correct because e-mails can serve as evidence. Likewise, options c and d are incorrect because they too may serve as evidence. Option b is incorrect because electronic information must not only be included but, for many providers (especially hospitals such as is the case here), it is the medium on which the vast majority of information about a patient resides (Rinehart-Thompson 2020, 57–58).

46. **a**   Common practice for covered entities is to accept the request, but not to agree to the restrictions because of the legal implications to the covered entity should the restriction be violated. Instead, if there are valid reasons why the patient requests the restriction, covered entities implement steps in an attempt to restrict the information as best as their systems and processes allow. The covered entity responds to the patient by describing measures it has taken but does not guarantee that the information is protected against incidental or accidental disclosure (Thomason 2013, 106–107).

47. **d**   A strategy included in a good security program is an employee security awareness program. Employees are often responsible for threats to data security. Consequently, employee awareness is a particularly important tool in reducing security breaches (Reynolds and Brodnik 2017a, 274).

48. **d**   Redisclosure is the process of releasing health record documentation originally created by a different provider. Federal and state regulations provide specific redisclosure guidelines. When in doubt, follow the same release and disclosure guidelines for other types of health information (Fahrenholz 2017b, 106).

49. **c**   The Privacy Rule introduced the standard that individuals should be informed of how covered entities use or disclose protected health information (PHI). This notice must be provided to an individual at his or her first contact with the covered entity (Rinehart-Thompson 2017c, 219).

50. **a**   There are circumstances in which PHI can be used or disclosed without the individual's written authorization and for which the individual does not have the opportunity to agree or object. These would include use and disclosure of medical information for treatment, payment, and operations. Utilization review is use of the information for operations. Sending records to a physician for continuity of care would be for treatment purposes (Rinehart-Thompson 2017c, 225–226).

51. **b**   The Privacy Rule lists two circumstances where protected health information (PHI) can be used or disclosed without the individual's authorization (although the individual must be informed in advance and given an opportunity to agree or object). One of these circumstances is disclosing PHI to a family member or a close friend that is directly relevant to his or her involvement with the patient's care or payment. Likewise, a covered entity may disclose PHI, including the patient's location, general condition, or death, to notify or assist in the notification of a family member, personal representative, or some other person responsible for the patient's care (Rinehart-Thompson 2017c, 225–226).

Domain 3 *Data Analytics and Informatics*

52. **b**   A closed system is one where all parts operate together without external influences. In an open system, the parts are affected by the environment (Amatayakul 2017, 32).

53. **c**   Identification of need is one of phases of the modern system development life cycle (SDCL). One of the components of this phase is performing change management to address the human factor elements (Amatayakul 2017, 46-47).

54. **a**   This model shows that the relationship between the data table (or entity) hospital and the data table (or entity) division is one-to-many. A one-to-many relationship means that for every instance of hospital stored in the database, many related instances of division may be stored. Reading the diagram in the other direction, each instance of division stored in the database is related to only one instance of hospital (Sayles and Kavanaugh-Burke 2021, 47-48).

55. **c**   In data mining, the analyst performs exploratory data analysis to determine trends and identify patterns in the data set (White 2020b, 520).

56. **d**   The record locator service (RLS) provides the ability to identify where records are located based on registered information about a person (Lee-Eichenwald 2020, 397–398).

57. **c**   The normal distribution is actually a theoretical family of distributions that may have any mean or any standard deviation. It is bell-shaped and symmetrical about the mean. Because it is symmetrical, 50 percent of the observations fall above the mean and 50 percent fall below it. In a normal distribution, the mean, median, and mode are equal (White 2020b, 512).

58. **c**   Clinical decision support systems refer to software that processes information to help users make a clinical decision. Clinical decision support systems can identify a potential problem (for example, a drug interaction or drug allergy) and issue an alert or a reminder that includes a recommendation for specific corrected action (Amatayakul 2017, 22–23).

59. **c**   Data mining is a technique of data analytics where the analyst determines any trends and identifies patterns in the data (White 2020b, 520).

60. **d**   Complaints such as "too many alerts" should not be dismissed because the frustration caused by the problem can lead to other issues exacerbating the results. On the other hand, taking immediate action to eliminate some of the alerts also poses risk that some important alerts will not be provided. Retraining one professional is also not likely to improve that individual's complaint, especially since it is likely many professionals have the same complaint. Instead, a formal data quality discovery process should be set up to evaluate and take corrective action relative to what we now call alert fatigue, or whatever other frequent complaint occurs (Amatayakul 2020, 437).

61. **b**   The patient meets severity of illness with the persistent fever and intensity of service with the inpatient-approved surgery scheduled within 24 hours of admission (Shaw and Carter 2019, 143).

62. **d**   A line graph or plot may be used to display time trends. The *x*-axis shows the unit of time from left to right, and the *y*-axis measures the values of the variable being plotted (Marc 2020, 537).

63. **a** Data are only meaningful in context. They must be formatted, filtered, and manipulated to be transformed into information and knowledge that can be acted on for decision-making in PI programs. In this scenario, the PI team did not provide the context regarding the data to administration in their presentation. These UTIs could have been HAIs, or patients could have been admitted to the facility with the UTI, so administration does not know why they should be concerned (Shaw and Carter 2019, 348).

64. **c** Relationships between objects and attributes help an information system achieve its purpose. Relationships tie the component parts together in accordance with their characteristics (Amatayatul 2017, 42).

65. **c** The sample migration path includes the applications of SDOH and population health. An operational element that should also be in place should be determining how SDOH will be collected and used (Amatayakul 2020, 416–418).

66. **d** In this situation there are too many changes occurring at the same time to determine what is improving the nursing staffing satisfaction scores. Any one item could be the reason for the improvement. To evaluate the impact of the electronic health record (EHR) nursing documentation component, a benefits realization study should have been utilized. This would have studied the impact of the EHR component before and after implementation (Amatayakul 2017, 106).

67. **b** Implementation of acquired health IT includes product installation, customization of the system to meet the organization's requirements, and turning the system over to users. It is important to recognize that implementation is more than just installation. A common misconception relating to EHR implementation is that software can be installed and used directly thereafter. Even the simplest EHR requires some system configuration, training, and testing (Amayatakul 2017, 49).

68. **d** A gross autopsy rate is the proportion or percentage of deaths that are followed by the performance of autopsy. Using this data, five patients had autopsies performed out of the 25 deaths; therefore, $5/25 = 0.2 \times 100 = 20\%$ (Edgerton 2020, 489).

69. **c** The mode is used to indicate the most frequent observation in a frequency distribution. In this data set there are three occurrences of the value 8 and only two or less occurrences of any other value, so 8 is the mode (Edgerton 2020, 477–478).

70. **c** Predictive modeling is a process used to identify patterns that can be used to predict the odds of a particular outcome based on the observed data. Predictive models use historical data in order to predict what is likely to happen in the future. For example, it might be used to predict the number of inpatient beds needed (White 2020b, 520-521).

71. **a** Alerts and reminders are provided to the physician or other healthcare provider as data are entered, thus identifying problems and key information at the point of capture rather than after review by nurses, pharmacists, or others. These alerts and reminders are controlled by clinical decision support built into the system, which is able to help prevent medication errors and improve the quality of care through its validation mechanisms (Sayles and Kavanaugh-Burke 2021, 171-172).

72. **b** The ICU bed count in the state has realized a decrease of 20%. Bed count is a component needed to calculate occupancy rates for any facility. In this situation the reduction of ICU beds at any healthcare facility in the state has the potential to increase the volume of patients in this hospital's ICU (Edgerton 2020, 483).

73. **c**   The Federated—inconsistent databases—model for HIE includes multiple enterprises agreeing to connect and share specific information in a point-to-point manner (Amatayakul 2017, 417–418).

74. **d**   A basic service provided by an HIE organization must be the actual transmission of the data, which is the technical networking service that provides appropriate bandwidth, latency, availability, ubiquity, and security (Amatayakul 2017, 420).

75. **b**   One way to describe all of the elements of an information system is to consider not only the hardware and software but also people, policy, and process. Policy refers to the directives or principles on which people perform their work or other activities. This cannot be overlooked when implementing health IT (Amatayakul 2017, 42).

76. **a**   Interoperability is the ability of different information technology systems and software applications to communicate; to exchange data accurately, effectively, and consistently; and to use the information that has been exchanged (Sayles and Kavanaugh-Burke 2021, 252).

77. **a**   Information warehouses allow organizations to store reports, presentations, profiles, and graphics interpreted and developed from stores of data for reuse in subsequent organizational activities (Shaw and Carter 2019, 350).

78. **a**   Algorithms are used by healthcare facilities and are relatively short computer programs of rules or procedures containing conditional logic for solving a problem or accomplishing a task. There are also guideline algorithms concerning rules for evaluating patient care against published guidelines (Sayles and Kavanaugh-Burke 2021, 158).

79. **b**   Character and symbol recognition technologies include bar coding, optical character recognition, and gesture recognition technologies. The bar code symbol was standardized for the healthcare industry, making it easier to adopt barcoding technology. Barcoding applications have been adopted for labels, patient wristbands, specimen containers, business/employee/patient records, library reference materials, medication packages, dietary items, paper documents, and more (Lee-Eichenwald 2020, 362).

80. **d**   One consequence of the proprietary nature of health IT systems has been that healthcare delivery organizations acquire one vendor's software to initiate their use of health IT and then find themselves dependent on the first vendor to meet all of their information system needs. Thus, proprietary systems that essentially force an organization to stay with one vendor have been the norm in the health IT marketplace. As time has gone on, however, the proprietary systems have become a huge barrier to exchanging health information among organizations and to reporting patient safety issues with the clinical decision support components (Amatayakul 2017, 33).

81. **d**   The clinician or physician web portals were first seen as a way for clinicians to easily access (via a web browser) the healthcare provider organizations' multiple sources of structured and unstructured data from any network-connected device. Like clinical workstations, clinician or physician web portals evolved into an effective medium for providing access to multiple applications as well as the data (Lee-Eichenwald 2020, 365).

82. **b**   Bar graphs are used to display data from one or more variables. The bars may be drawn vertically or horizontally. Bar graphs are used for nominal or ordinal variables. In this case, you would be displaying the average length of stay by service and then within each service have a bar for each hospital (White 2020a, 209).

83. **d**   Predictive modeling applies statistical techniques to determine the likelihood of certain events occurring together. Statistical methods are applied to historical data to learn the patterns in the data. These patterns are used to create models of what is most likely to occur (White 2021, 10; White 2020b, 521).

84. **b**   Contingency tables are a useful method for displaying the relationship between two categorical variables. Contingency tables are often referred to by the number of rows and columns (White 2021, 75).

85. **c**   The systems development life cycle (SDLC) phase of maintenance relates to the ongoing support needed to keep the system current and accurate. As part of this phase out-of-date system components are disposed of (Amatayakul 2017, 49).

Domain 4   *Revenue Cycle Management*

86. **c**   Unbundling is the practice of using multiple codes that describe individual components of a procedure rather than using an appropriate single code that describes all steps of the procedure performed. Unbundling is a component of the NCCI and is what the coder in this example was doing. The use of audits or other evaluation techniques to monitor compliance and assist in the reduction of identified problem areas and corporate compliance is necessary to become aware of coding issues and stop them. The coder would need to be educated regarding unbundling and would be advised to stop the practice immediately (Huey 2021, 409).

87. **b**   A bill cannot be generated until the coding is complete, so organizations routinely monitor the discharged, not final billed (DNFB) days. Generally, this is done by reviewing the DNFB report that includes all patients who have been discharged from the facility, but for whom the billing process is not complete (Handlon 2020, 253).

88. **b**   Each diagnosis-related group (DRG) is assigned a relative weight (RW). The RW is a multiplier that determines reimbursement. For example, a DRG with a relative weight of 2.0000 would pay twice as much as a DRG with a RW of 1.0000 (Hazelwood 2020, 229).

89. **a**   The patient has esophageal reflux with no esophagitis mentioned, therefore K21.9 is the correct diagnosis code. For the ICD-10-PCS procedure code, a closed biopsy of the esophagus was performed via esophagoscopy and therefore 0DB58ZX is the correct code. The Section is Medical and Surgical—character 0; Body System is Gastrointestinal—character D; Root Operation is Excision—character B; Body Part is Esophagus—character 5; Approach—Via a Natural or Artificial Opening Endoscopic—character 8; No Device—character Z; and the procedure was for diagnostic reasons—character X (Schraffenberger and Palkie 2022, 43–44; Kuehn and Jorwic 2023, 30, 76-78).

90. **c**   Care Compare, formerly known as Hospital Compare, reports on measures of hospital quality of care for heart attack, heart failure, pneumonia, and the prevention of surgical infections. The data available is available at the Medicare.gov website. (White 2021, 34-35).

91. **a**   The hospital value-based purchasing (VBP) will measure hospital performance using four domains. The domain scores are combined resulting in a total performance score (TPS). A facility's TPS determines what portion of the hold back amount the facility will earn back. For every point increase in the TPS, the provider will increase payment by a portion of the hold back dollars, so in this VBP, the higher TPS score is desired (Casto and White 2021, 83-84).

92. **d** Medical identity theft occurs when a patient uses another person's name and insurance information to receive healthcare benefits. Most often this is done so a person can receive medical care with an insurance benefit and pay less or nothing for the care he or she receives (Rinehart-Thompson 2020, 67).

93. **a** The health insurance policy coverage includes legally married spouses, children and young adults until they reach age 26. The definition of children includes natural children, legally adopted children, stepchildren, and children who are dependent during the waiting period before adoption, but would not necessarily include everyone in the household (Casto and White 2021, 19).

94. **a** Newly insured and Medicaid-eligible patients would have potentially been heavily discounted self-pay or charity care prior to entering the exchanges. Therefore, providers will likely have fewer losses due to uncollectible debt and uncompensated care (Davis and Doyle 2016, 68–69).

95. **d** In conjunction with the corporate compliance officer, the health information manager should provide education and training related to the importance of complete and accurate coding, documentation, and billing on an annual basis. Technical education for all coders should be provided. Documentation education is also part of compliance education. A focused effort should be made to provide documentation education to the medical staff. Coding is based primarily on physician documentation, so nursing staff would not be included in the education process (Hunt and Kirk 2020, 298).

96. **c** Aging of accounts is maintained in 30-day increments (0–30 days, 31–60 days, and so forth) (Casto and White 2021, 170).

97. **d** When the claim is submitted the reviewer should compare all the diagnoses and procedures printed on the bill with the coded information in the health record system. This process will help identify whether the communication software between the health record system and the billing system is functioning correctly. The HIM department should share the results of this comparison with patient financial services and the information technology department (Casto and White 2021, 168).

98. **a** A query is a routine communication and education tool used to advocate for complete and compliant documentation. The query is directed to the provider who originated the progress note or other report in question. This could include the attending physician, consulting physician, or the surgeon. In most cases, a query for abnormal test results would be directed to the attending physician (Hunt and Kirk 2020, 285–287).

99. **b** Nonparticipating providers (nonPARs) do not sign a participation agreement with Medicare but may or may not accept assignment. If the nonPAR physician elects to accept assignment, he or she is paid 95 percent (5 percent less than participating physicians). For example, if the MFS amount is $200, the PAR provider receives $160 (80 percent of $200), but the nonPAR provider receives only $152 (95 percent of $160). In this case, the physician is participating so he or she will receive 80 percent of the MFS or $240 (80 percent of $300) (Casto and White 2021, 125).

100. **c** Begin with the main term of hernia repair; inguinal; incarcerated. The age of the patient and the fact that the hernia is not recurrent make the choice 49507 (Huey 2021, 24, 152-154).

101. **d** The urinary tract infection (UTI) would be coded as present on admission (POA) as the symptoms of the UTI were documented by the provider in the emergency room prior to admission. Conditions that develop during an outpatient encounter, including in the emergency department are considered POA (Hazelwood 2020, 230–231).

102. **b**   Standards of care are not defined in NCDs and LCDs. LCDs and NCDs are limited to certain procedures and services, but not all services and procedures provided to patients. LCDs and NCDs directly impact whether payment is made if specified conditions are not met (Handlon 2020, 247–248).

103. **a**   The focused review indicated areas of risk related to lower weighted MS-DRGs from triple and pair combinations which may be the result of a coder missing secondary diagnoses. A focused audit based on this specific potential problem area could help to identify these cases. Optimization seeks the most accurate documentation, coded data, and resulting payment in the amount the provider is rightly and legally entitled to receive (Schraffenberger and Kuehn 2011, 314–315).

104. **a**   As part of the move to pay for value, CMS developed their value-based purchasing (VBP) program as part of the Affordable Care Act. This VBP program includes four domains: safety, clinical care, efficiency and cost reduction, and person and community engagement. Each domain includes a variety of measures that must be reported to CMS regularly. Catheter-associated UTIs and surgical site infections are part of the Safety Domain of the VBP program (Shaw and Carter 2019, 135–136).

105. **d**   It is not appropriate for the coder to assume that the removal was done by either snare, ablation, or hot biopsy forceps. The coding professional must query the physician to assign the appropriate code (Hunt and Kirk 2020, 285–287).

106. **d**   Forms of prospective reimbursement are capitation, case-rate global payment, and bundled payment. The capitated payment method, or capitation, is a method of payment for health services in which the third-party payer reimburses providers a fixed, per capita amount for a period. "Per capita" means "per head" or "per person" (Casto and White 2021, 54-55).

107. **b**   Main term: Depression, subterm: recurrent; see Disorder, depressive, recurrent. Follow the cross reference to Disorder, depressive, recurrent, severe F33.2 (Schraffenberger and Palkie 2022, 43–44).

108. **c**   Late charges are any charges that have not been posted to the account number within the healthcare facility's established bill hold time period. By incorporating this predicted billing delay into normal operations, the facility creates a preventive control to avoid under billing or having to submit late charges to the payer. For the provider to be paid for these charges, an adjusted claim must be sent to Medicare (Handlon 2020, 255).

109. **c**   Once the claim is submitted to the third-party payer for reimbursement, the accounts receivable clock begins (Casto and White 2021, 170).

110. **a**   Verifying payment received is reflective of payment agreements to identify discrepancies in term application or interpretation (Handlon 2020, 265).

111. **b**   Hospitals have invested in clinical documentation improvement (CDI) programs to assure the health record accurately reflects the actual condition of the patient. Some of the goals of a CDI program include: identifying and clarifying missing, conflicting, or nonspecific physician documentation related to diagnosis and procedures; promoting health record completion during the patient's course of care; and improving communication between physicians and other members of the healthcare team (Hunt and Kirk 2020, 276).

112. **a**   In the outpatient setting, do not code a diagnosis documented as "probable." Rather, code the conditions to the highest degree of certainty for the encounter (Schraffenberger and Palkie 2022, 105).

113. **b**   To determine the appropriate MS-DRG, a claim for a healthcare encounter is first classified into one of 25 major diagnostic categories (MDCs). The principal diagnosis determines the MDC assignment. The principal diagnosis is the condition established after study to have resulted in the inpatient admission (Casto and White 2021, 76).

114.. **b**   Focused selections of coded accounts are necessary for deeper understanding of patterns of error or change in high-risk areas or other areas of specific concern. Optimization seeks the most accurate documentation, coded data, and resulting payment in the amount the provider is rightly and legally entitled to receive (Schraffenberger and Kuehn 2011, 271).

115. **c**   During a clinical documentation improvement quality review, an organization should track and monitor the following elements: validity of queries generated, validity of working DRG assignment, validity of CDI specialist's assignment, and missed query opportunities (Hess 2015, 210).

116. **a**   Preregistration, which occurs in the front-end process, includes confirming eligibility and insurance benefits (Handlon 2020, 246).

117. **a**   In many instances, patients have more than one insurance policy and the determination of which policy is primary and which is secondary is necessary so that there is no duplication in payment of benefits. This process is called coordination of benefits (COB) (Casto and White 2021, 24-25).

Domain 5   *Management and Leadership*

118. **d**   Change management can be best described as the formal process of introducing change, getting it adopted, and diffusing it throughout the organization (Kelly and Greenstone 2020, 87).

119. **a**   In peer review, a member of a profession assesses the work of colleagues within that same profession. Peer review has traditionally been at the center of quality assessment and assurance efforts. The medical profession's peer review efforts have emphasized the scientific aspects of quality. Appropriate use of pharmaceuticals, postoperative infection rates, and accuracy of diagnosis are among the measures of quality that have been used. Peer review is a requirement of both CMS and the Joint Commission (Fuller 2020, 27).

120. **a**   Knowledge of the internal and external environment is essential to vision and strategy formulation. An environmental assessment is defined as a thorough review of the internal and external conditions in which an organization operates. This data-intensive process is the continuous process of gathering and analyzing intelligence about trends that are—or may be— affecting an organization and industry. IBM did not see the market demands and change in the personal home computing environment quickly enough, so their competitors were out to market ahead of them (McClernon 2020, 921).

121. **c**   Performance measurement in healthcare provides an indication of an organization's performance in relation to a specified process or outcome. An outcome measure may be the effect of care, treatment, or services on a customer (Shaw and Carter 2019, 41).

122. **a**   A permanent variance is a financial term that refers to the difference between the budgeted amount and the actual amount of a line item that is not expected to reverse itself during a subsequent period (Revoir 2020, 834).

123. **a**   Every aspect of management involves a strategic management component. With organizational learning as a centerpiece, this approach unifies change management, strategy development, and leadership. In all three, people learn by observing and reflecting on the results of experiences (McClernon 2020, 918).

124. **c**   DURSA is a legally binding contract defining the requirements for participation in the eHealthExchange national network (Lee-Eichenwald 2020, 396).

125. **c**   Ground rules must be agreed upon by the team at the very beginning of the process improvement effort. All members of the team should have input into the ground rules. They should agree to abide by them for the sake of the team's success (Shaw and Carter 2019, 59).

126. **c**   Strategic planning is a formalized roadmap that describes how the company executes the chosen strategy. A strategic plan spells out where an organization is going over the next three to five years and how it is going to get there. HIM professionals can use strategy to shape and influence change in their department and organization (McClernon 2020, 916).

127. **d**   The discipline of ergonomics has helped redefine the employee workspace with consideration for comfort and safety (Oachs 2020, 763).

128. **c**   Blood-borne pathogens, such as HIV and hepatitis B and C, are transported through contact with infected body fluids such as blood, semen, and vomitus. Each facility should define the employee level of risk for infection associated with their job classification and define the proper precautions needed to prevent exposure. Most healthcare facilities require employee job descriptions to carry a definition of blood-borne pathogen risk associated with the job task (Shaw and Carter 2019, 179).

129. **c**   Medicare certification and the ability of a healthcare provider to participate in the Medicaid program is based on an annual unannounced survey conducted by a state agency that has contracted to act on behalf of CMS (Rinehart-Thompson 2017e, 253).

130. **d**   Conflict management focuses on working with the individuals involved to find a mutually acceptable solution. There are three ways to address conflict: compromise, control, and constructive confrontation. Constructive confrontation is a method in which both parties meet with an objective third party to explore their perceptions and feelings. The desired outcome is to produce a mutual understanding of the issues and to create a win-win situation (LeBlanc 2020, 713).

131. **a**   The Hay Guide Chart-Profile Method of Job Evaluation is widely used as a job evaluation tool (LeBlanc 2020, 709–710).

132. **b**   The elements of a contract must be stated clearly and specifically. A contract cannot exist unless all the following elements exist: there must be an agreement between two or more persons or entities and the agreement must include a valid offer, acceptance, and exchange of consideration (Rinehart-Thompson 2020, 54).

133. **d**   People exhibit the bandwagon effect when they do something simply because other people are doing it (Kelly and Greenstone 2020, 49).

134. **c**   SWOT analysis looks at the internal strengths of an organization or department, and the external opportunities and threats. These are considered to be elements that the department can control. In this scenario there is an opportunity that is created for the organization as new coders will be available based on the HIM program that is found in the community (Kelly and Greenstone 2020, 30–31).

135. **d**   The on-site survey for the Joint Commission utilizes a tracer methodology that permits assessment of operational systems and processes in relation to the actual experiences of selected patients currently under the organization's care. Tracer methodology analyzes an organization's systems, with particular attention to identified priority focus areas, by following individual patients through the organization's healthcare process in the sequence experienced by its patients (Shaw and Carter 2019, 335).

136. **b**   The net income is based only on the arithmetic difference between total revenue and total expenses of the current fiscal year. The difference between the total revenue of $2,500,000 and the total expenses of $2,250,000 is $250,000 (Revoir 2020, 821).

137. **d**   The difference between assets and liabilities is referred to as net assets. These relationships can be expressed in the following equation:

$$Assets - Liabilities = Net\ assets\ (equity)$$

In this example, add the assets (cash $500,000 + A/R $250,000 + building $1,000,000 + land $700,000 = $2,450,000) and then subtract the liabilities (A/P $350,000 + mortgage $600,000 = $950,000) or $2,450,000 – $950,000 = $1,500,000 (Revoir 2020, 814).

138. **b**   Job-knowledge questions are intended to determine if the applicant knows how to do the job (Kelly and Greenstone 2020, 164).

139. **b**   Work sampling is a statistical method that reviews a select portion of tasks performed and provides baseline data for further job performance assessment (Kelly and Greenstone 2020, 183).

140. **b**   Basic work distribution data can be collected in a work distribution chart, which is initially filled out by each employee and includes all responsible task content. Task content should come directly from the employee's current job description. In addition to task content, each employee tracks each task's start time, end time, and volume or productivity within a typical workweek. The results of a work distribution analysis can lead a department to redefine the job descriptions of some employees, redesign the office layout, or establish new or revised procedures for some department functions in order to gain improvements in staff productivity or service quality (Oachs 2020, 765).

141. **d**   Self-directed learning allows participants to control their learning and progress at their own pace. This delivery method supports adult learners who wish to have some control over when and where their learning takes place (Kelly and Greenstone 2020, 211).

142. **c**   Videoconferencing permits additional flexibility in delivering courses that may be enhanced through visual as well as audio presentation, such as those that include demonstrations or simulation exercises. Videoconferencing is useful for training employees in organizations with multiple sites, such as integrated delivery networks with inpatient and outpatient facilities. The expense is justified for large organizations that do extensive training (Patena 2020, 747).

143. **a** Every accreditation, certification, and licensure agency develops written standards or regulations that serve as the basis of the review process. It is imperative that healthcare facilities monitor any changes and updates to the various standards and regulations and keep current sets of them on hand at all times to help maintain compliance status. Compliance is the process of meeting a prescribed set of standards or regulations to maintain active accreditation, licensure, or certification status (Shaw and Carter 2019, 330).

144. **a** Standards that are measurable and relevant to an employee's overall performance are helpful in setting clear expectations. They also are useful in providing constructive feedback (LeBlanc 2020, 701).

145. **b** Simulation provides real-world situations that represent the actual situation, such a natural disaster. This allows learners to react to a situation in a hands-on way. Diversity training, annual coding updates, and new employee orientation are better suited for a classroom or a similar type of delivery method (Kelly and Greenstone 2020, 211).

146. **a** A request for proposal (RFP) would be the first step at this point as the organization has determined a new vendor is needed. An RFP is a solicitation to vendors that includes and organization's requirements for functionality, vendor strategy, and other elements being sought from a vendor, and that usually also includes basic information about the healthcare organization, such a how many users will be using the system, the timeline for implementation, and any special contractual issues that must be addressed (Lee-Eichenwald 2020, 396).

147. **c** Off-site seminars are more expensive than on-site learning. They can be cost effective if more than one individual is being trained, but seminars are expensive (Kelly and Greenstone 2020, 212).

148. **d** Credentialing is the process that requires the verification of the educational qualifications, licensure status, and other experience of healthcare professionals who have applied for the privilege of practicing within a healthcare facility (Fahrenholz 2017b, 79–80).

149. **d** Responses a, b, and c represent inputs into the project whereas response d is the output from the project (Olson 2020, 851–853).

150. **a** When a manager is planning to contract for staffing in a transitional situation in order to meet organizational goals, various types of contracts can be considered. In this situation, a temporary contract would be used. Contracting for staff to cover for a temporary situation in order to keep productivity in line is a temporary contract (Oachs 2020, 769).

RESOURCES

References

Primary References

AHIMA (American Health Information Management Association). 2017. *Pocket Glossary of Health Information Management and Technology,* 5th ed. Chicago: AHIMA.

Amatayakul, M.K. 2020. "Health Information Systems Strategic Planning." Chapter 13 in *Health Information Management: Concepts, Principles, and Practice,* 6th ed., edited by P. Oachs and A. Watters. Chicago: AHIMA.

Amatayakul, M.K. 2017. *Health IT and EHRs: Principles and Practice,* 6th ed. Chicago: AHIMA.

Biedermann, S. and D. Dolezel. 2017. *Introduction to Healthcare Informatics,* 2nd ed. Chicago: AHIMA.

Bowman, S. 2017. "Corporate Compliance." Chapter 18 in *Fundamentals of Law for Health Informatics and Information Management*, 3rd ed., edited by M.S. Brodnik, L.A. Rinehart-Thompson, and R.B. Reynolds. Chicago: AHIMA.

Brinda, D. and A.L. Watters. 2020. "Data Privacy, Confidentiality, and Security." Chapter 11 in *Health Information Management: Concepts, Principles, and Practice,* 6th ed., edited by P. Oachs and A. Watters. Chicago: AHIMA.

Brodnik, M.S. 2017a. "Introduction to the Fundamentals of Law for Health Informatics and Information Management." Chapter 1 in *Fundamentals of Law for Health Informatics and Information Management*, 3rd ed., edited by M.S. Brodnik, L.A. Rinehart-Thompson, and R.B. Reynolds. Chicago: AHIMA.

Brodnik, M.S. 2017b. "Access, Use, and Disclosure and Release of Health Information." Chapter 15 in *Fundamentals of Law for Health Informatics and Information Management*, 3rd ed., edited by M.S. Brodnik, L.A. Rinehart-Thompson, and R.B. Reynolds. Chicago: AHIMA.

Brodnik, M.S. 2017c. "Required Reporting and Mandatory Disclosure Laws." Chapter 16 in *Fundamentals of Law for Health Informatics and Information Management*, 3rd ed., edited by M.S. Brodnik, L.A. Rinehart-Thompson, and R.B. Reynolds. Chicago: AHIMA.

Brodnik, M.S., L.A. Rinehart-Thompson, and R.B. Reynolds. 2017. *Fundamentals of Law for Health Informatics and Information Management*, 3rd ed. Chicago: AHIMA.

Casto, A.B. and S. White. 2021. *Principles of Healthcare Reimbursement,* 7th ed. Chicago: AHIMA. Davis, N. and B. Doyle. 2016. *Revenue Cycle Management Best Practices,* 2nd ed. Chicago, IL: American Health Information Management Association.

Edgerton, C. 2020. "Healthcare Statistics." Chapter 15 in *Health Information Management: Concepts, Principles, and Practice,* 6th ed., edited by P. Oachs and A. Watters. Chicago: AHIMA.

Fahrenholz, C.G. 2017a. "Clinical Documentation and the Health Record." Chapter 2 in *Documentation for Health Records,* 2nd ed., edited by C.G. Fahrenholz. Chicago: AHIMA.

Fahrenholz, C.G. 2017b. "Principal and Ancillary Functions of the Healthcare Record." Chapter 3 in *Documentation for Health Records,* 2nd ed., edited by C.G. Fahrenholz. Chicago: AHIMA.

Fahrenholz, C.G. 2017c. "Documentation for Statistical Reporting and Public Health." Chapter 4 in *Documentation for Health Records,* 2nd ed., edited by C.G. Fahrenholz. Chicago: AHIMA.

Fahrenholz, C.G. 2017d. "Healthcare Delivery." Chapter 1 in *Documentation for Health Records,* 2nd ed., edited by C.G. Fahrenholz. Chicago: AHIMA.

Fahrenholz, C.G. 2017e. "Healthcare Delivery." Introduction in *Documentation for Health Records,* 2nd ed., edited by C.G. Fahrenholz. Chicago: AHIMA.

Fahrenholz, C.G. ed. 2017. *Documentation for Health Records,* 2nd ed. Chicago: AHIMA.

Fuller, S.R. 2020. "The US Healthcare Delivery System." Chapter 1 in *Health Information Management: Concepts, Principles, and Practice,* 6th ed., edited by P. Oachs and A. Watters. Chicago: AHIMA.

Glondys, B.A. and L. Kadlec. 2017. "EHRs Serving as the Business and Legal Records of Healthcare Organizations" (2016 Update). Appendix 3B in *Documentation for Health Records,* 2nd ed., edited by C.G. Fahrenholz. Chicago: AHIMA.

Handlon, L. 2020. "Revenue Cycle Management." Chapter 8 in *Health Information Management: Concepts, Principles, and Practice,* 6th ed., edited by P. Oachs and A. Watters. Chicago: AHIMA.

Hazelwood, A.C. 2020. "Reimbursement Methodologies." Chapter 7 in *Health Information Management: Concepts, Principles, and Practice,* 6th ed., edited by P. Oachs and A. Watters. Chicago: AHIMA.

Hess, P. 2015. *Clinical Documentation Improvement: Principles and Practice.* Chicago: AHIMA.

Houser, S. 2020. "Research Methods." Chapter 18 in *Health Information Management: Concepts, Principles, and Practice,* 6th ed., edited by P. Oachs and A. Watters. Chicago: AHIMA.

Huey, K. 2021. *Procedural Coding and Reimbursement for Physician Services: Applying Current Procedural Terminology and HCPCS 2021.* Chicago: AHIMA.

Hunt, T. J. and K. Kirk. 2020. "Clinical Documentation Integrity and Coding Compliance." Chapter 9 in *Health Information Management: Concepts, Principles, and Practice,* 6th ed., edited by P. Oachs and A. Watters. Chicago: AHIMA.

Hunt, T. J. 2017. "Clinical Documentation Improvement." Chapter 6 in *Documentation for Health Records,* 2nd ed., edited by C.G. Fahrenholz. Chicago: AHIMA.

James, E.L. 2017a. "Long-Term Care Hospitals." Chapter 11 in *Documentation for Health Records,* 2nd ed., edited by C.G. Fahrenholz. Chicago: AHIMA.

James, E.L. 2017b. "Facility-Based Long-Term Care." Chapter 12 in *Documentation for Health Records,* 2nd ed., edited by C.G. Fahrenholz. Chicago: AHIMA.

Jenkins, N.R. 2017. "Clinical Information and Nonclinical Data, Health Record Design." Chapter 5 in *Documentation for Health Records,* 2nd ed., edited by C.G. Fahrenholz. Chicago: AHIMA.

Johns, M. 2020. "Data Governance and Stewardship." Chapter 3 in *Health Information Management: Concepts, Principles, and Practice,* 6th ed., edited by P. Oachs and A. Watters. Chicago: AHIMA.

Johns, M. 2015. *Enterprise Health Information Management and Data Governance.* Chicago: AHIMA.

Kelly, J. and P. Greenstone. 2020. *Management of the Health Information Professional,* 2nd ed. Chicago: AHIMA.

Klaver, J.C. 2017a. "Evidence." Chapter 5 in *Fundamentals of Law for Health Informatics and Information Management,* 3rd ed., edited by M.S. Brodnik, L.A. Rinehart-Thompson, and R.B. Reynolds. Chicago: AHIMA.

Klaver, J.C. 2017b. "Corporations, Contracts, and Antitrust Legal Issues." Chapter 7 in *Fundamentals of Law for Health Informatics and Information Management,* 3rd ed., edited by M.S. Brodnik, L.A. Rinehart-Thompson, and R.B. Reynolds. Chicago: AHIMA.

Klaver, J.C. 2017c. "Consent to Treatment." Chapter 8 in *Fundamentals of Law for Health Informatics and Information Management,* 3rd ed., edited by M.S. Brodnik, L.A. Rinehart-Thompson, and R.B. Reynolds. Chicago: AHIMA.

Kuehn, L.M. and T.M. Jorwic. 2023. *ICD-10-PCS An Applied Approach 2023.* Chicago: AHIMA.

LeBlanc, M.M. 2020. "Human Resource Management." Chapter 22 in *Health Information Management: Concepts, Principles, and Practice,* 6th ed., edited by P. Oachs and A. Watters. Chicago: AHIMA.

Lee-Eichenwald, S. 2020. "Health Information Technologies." Chapter 12 in *Health Information Management: Concepts, Principles, and Practice,* 6th ed., edited by P. Oachs and A. Watters. Chicago: AHIMA

Marc, D. 2020. "Data Visualization." Chapter 17 in *Health Information Management: Concepts, Principles, and Practice,* 6th ed., edited by P. Oachs and A. Watters. Chicago: AHIMA.

McClernon, S.E. 2020. "Strategic Thinking and Management." Chapter 28 in *Health Information Management: Concepts, Principles, and Practice,* 6th ed., edited by P. Oachs and A. Watters. Chicago: AHIMA.

Oachs, P.K. 2020. "Work Design and Process Improvement." Chapter 24 in *Health Information Management: Concepts, Principles, and Practice,* 6th ed., edited by P. Oachs and A. Watters. Chicago: AHIMA.

Oachs, P.K. and A.L. Watters, eds. 2020. *Health Information Management: Concepts, Principles, and Practice,* 6th ed. Chicago: AHIMA.

O'Dell, R.M. 2020 "Quality Management." Chapter 20 in *Health Information Management: Concepts, Principles, and Practice,* 6th ed., edited by P. Oachs and A. Watters. Chicago: AHIMA.

Olenik, K. and R.B. Reynolds. 2017. "Security Threats and Controls." Chapter 13 in *Fundamentals of Law for Health Informatics and Information Management*, 3rd ed., edited by M.S. Brodnik, L.A. Rinehart-Thompson, and R.B. Reynolds. Chicago: AHIMA.

Olson, B.D. 2020. "Project Management." Chapter 26 in *Health Information Management: Concepts, Principles, and Practice*, 6th ed., edited by P. Oachs and A. Watters. Chicago: AHIMA.Palkie, B. 2020a. "Clinical Classifications, Vocabularies, Terminologies, and Standards." Chapter 5 in *Health Information Management: Concepts, Principles, and Practice*, 6th ed., edited by P. Oachs and A. Watters. Chicago: AHIMA.

Palkie, B. 2020a. "Clinical Classifications, Vocabularies, Terminologies, and Standards." Chapter 5 in *Health Information Management: Concepts, Principles, and Practice*, 6th ed., edited by P. Oachs and A. Watters. Chicago: AHIMA.

Palkie, B. 2020b. "Organizational Compliance and Risk." Chapter 10 in *Health Information Management: Concepts, Principles, and Practice,* 6th ed., edited by P. Oachs and A. Watters. Chicago: AHIMA.

Patena, K.R. 2020. "Employee Training and Development." Chapter 23 in *Health Information Management: Concepts, Principles, and Practice,* 6th ed., edited by P. Oachs and A. Watters. Chicago: AHIMA.

Revoir, R. 2020. "Financial Management." Chapter 25 in *Health Information Management: Concepts, Principles, and Practice,* 6th ed., edited by P. Oachs and A. Watters. Chicago: AHIMA.

Reynolds, R.B. and M.S. Brodnik. 2017a. "The HIPAA Security Rule." Chapter 12 in *Fundamentals of Law for Health Informatics and Information Management*, 3rd ed., edited by M.S. Brodnik, L.A. Rinehart-Thompson, and R.B. Reynolds. Chicago: AHIMA.

Reynolds, R.B. and M.S. Brodnik. 2017b. "Medical Staff." Chapter 19 in *Fundamentals of Law for Health Informatics and Information Management*, 3rd ed., edited by M.S. Brodnik, L.A. Rinehart-Thompson, and R.B. Reynolds. Chicago: AHIMA.

Reynolds, R.B. and M.S. Brodnik. 2017c. "Workplace Law." Chapter 20 in *Fundamentals of Law for Health Informatics and Information Management*, 3rd ed., edited by M.S. Brodnik, L.A. Rinehart-Thompson, and R.B. Reynolds. Chicago: AHIMA.

Reynolds, R.B. and A. Morey. 2020. "Heath Record Content and Documentation." Chapter 4 in *Health Information Management: Concepts, Principles, and Practice,* 6th ed., edited by P. Oachs and A. Watters. Chicago: AHIMA.

Rinehart-Thompson, L.A. 2020. "Legal Issues in Health Information Management." Chapter 2 in *Health Information Management: Concepts, Principles, and Practice,* 6th ed., edited by P. Oachs and A. Watters. Chicago: AHIMA.

Rinehart-Thompson, L.A. 2018. *Introduction to Health Information Privacy and Security,* 2nd ed. Chicago: AHIMA.

Rinehart-Thompson, L.A. 2017a. "Legal Proceedings." Chapter 4 in *Fundamentals of Law for Health Informatics and Information Management*, 3rd ed., edited by M.S. Brodnik, L.A. Rinehart-Thompson, and R.B. Reynolds. Chicago: AHIMA.

Rinehart-Thompson, L.A. 2017b. "Legal Health Record: Maintenance, Content, Documentation, and Disposition." Chapter 9 in *Fundamentals of Law for Health Informatics and Information Management*, 3rd ed., edited by M.S. Brodnik, L.A. Rinehart-Thompson, and R.B. Reynolds. Chicago: AHIMA.

Rinehart-Thompson, L.A. 2017c. "HIPAA Privacy Rule: Part I." Chapter 10 in *Fundamentals of Law for Health Informatics and Information Management*, 3rd ed., edited by M.S. Brodnik, L.A. Rinehart-Thompson, and R.B. Reynolds. Chicago: AHIMA.

Rinehart-Thompson, L.A. 2017d. "HIPAA Privacy Rule: Part II." Chapter 11 in *Fundamentals of Law for Health Informatics and Information Management*, 3rd ed., edited by M.S. Brodnik, L.A. Rinehart-Thompson, and R.B. Reynolds. Chicago: AHIMA.

Rinehart-Thompson, L.A. 2017e. "Federal and State Requirements and Accreditation Guidelines." Chapter 9 in *Documentation for Health Records,* 2nd ed., edited by C.G. Fahrenholz. Chicago: AHIMA.

Sandefer, R.H. 2020. "Consumer Health Informatics." Chapter 14 in *Health Information Management: Concepts, Principles, and Practice,* 6th ed., edited by P. Oachs and A. Watters. Chicago: AHIMA.

Sayles, N.B. and L. Kavanaugh-Burke. 2021. *Introduction to Information Systems for Health Information Technology*, 4th ed. Chicago: AHIMA.

Schraffenberger, L.A. and L. Kuehn. 2011. *Effective Management of Coding Services,* 3rd ed. Chicago: AHIMA.

Schraffenberger, L.A. and B. Palkie. 2022. *Basic ICD-10-CM and ICD-10-PCS Coding, 2022*. Chicago: AHIMA.

Selman-Holman, L. 2017. "Home Care and Hospital Documentation, Liability, and Standards." Chapter 13 in *Documentation for Health Records,* 2nd ed., edited by C.G. Fahrenholz. Chicago: AHIMA.

Sharp, M.Y. and C. Madlock-Brown. 2020. "Data Management." Chapter 6 in *Health Information Management: Concepts, Principles, and Practice,* 6th ed., edited by P. Oachs and A. Watters. Chicago: AHIMA.

Shaw, P.L. and D. Carter. 2019. *Quality and Performance Improvement in Healthcare: Theory, Practice, and Management*, 7th ed. Chicago: AHIMA.

Swenson, D.X. 2020. "Managing and Leading during Organizational Change." Chapter 21 in *Health Information Management: Concepts, Principles, and Practice,* 6th ed., edited by P. Oachs and A. Watters. Chicago: AHIMA.

Swirsky, E.S. 2020. "Ethical Issues in Health Information." Chapter 27 in *Health Information Management: Concepts, Principles, and Practice,* 6th ed., edited by P. Oachs and A. Watters. Chicago: AHIMA.

Theodos, K. 2017. "Law and Ethics." Chapter 2 in *Fundamentals of Law for Health Informatics and Information Management*, 3rd ed., edited by M.S. Brodnik, L.A. Rinehart-Thompson, and R.B. Reynolds. Chicago: AHIMA.

Thomason, M.C. 2013. *HIPAA by Example: Application of Privacy Laws,* 2nd ed. Chicago: AHIMA.

White, S. 2021. *A Practical Approach to Analyzing Healthcare Data*, 4th ed. Chicago: AHIMA.

White, S. 2020a. *Calculating and Reporting Healthcare Statistics*, 6th ed. Chicago: AHIMA.

White, S. 2020b. "Healthcare Data Analytics." Chapter 16 in *Health Information Management: Concepts, Principles, and Practice,* 6th ed., edited by P. Oachs and A. Watters. Chicago: AHIMA.

Secondary References from Answer Key Rationales

45 CFR 160:103: General administrative requirements: General Provisions: Definitions. 2006.

45 CFR 164: 501: Uses and disclosures of protected health information (general rules). 2006.

45 CFR 164: 502b: Minimum necessary. 2006.

45 CFR 164: 506: Uses and disclosures for which authorization is required. 2006.

45 CFR 164: 508: Uses and disclosures for which authorization is required. 2006.

AHIMA (American Health Information Management Association). 2013 (January 25). Analysis of Modifications to the HIPAA Privacy, Security, Enforcement, and Breach Notification Rules under the Health Information Technology for Economic and Clinical Health Act and the Genetic Information Nondiscrimination Act; Other Modifications to the HIPAA Rules. http://bok.ahima.org/PdfView?oid=106127.

AHIMA (American Health Information Management Association). 2009 (February). Redisclosure of Patient Health Information (Updated). *Journal of AHIMA.* 80(2):51–54.

AMIA (American Medical Informatics Association). n.d. Consumer Health Informatics. https://www.amia.org/applications-informatics/consumer-health-informatics.

Rob, P. and C. Coronel. 2009. *Database Systems: Design, Implementation, and Management,* 8th ed. Boston, MA: Course Technology, Thomson Learning.

Robert, M. 2006. *The New Strategic Thinking: Pure and Simple.* New York: McGraw-Hill.

Hospital Statistical Formulas Used for the RHIA Exam

Hospital Statistical Formulas Used for the RHIA Exam

Average Daily Census

$$\frac{\text{Total service days for the unit for the period}}{\text{Total number of days in the period}}$$

Average Length of Stay

$$\frac{\text{Total length of stay (discharge days)}}{\text{Total discharges (includes deaths)}}$$

Percentage of Occupancy

$$\frac{\text{Total service days for a period}}{\text{Total bed count days in the period}} \times 100$$

Hospital Death Rate (Gross)

$$\frac{\text{Number of deaths of inpatients in period}}{\text{Number of discharges (including deaths)}} \times 100$$

Gross Autopsy Rate

$$\frac{\text{Total inpatient autopsies for a given period}}{\text{Total inpatient deaths for the period}} \times 100$$

Net Autopsy Rate

$$\frac{\text{Total inpatients for a given period}}{\text{Total inpatient deaths} - \text{unautopsied coroners' or medical examiners' cases}} \times 100$$

Hospital Autopsy Rate (Adjusted)

$$\frac{\text{Total hospital autopsies}}{\text{Number of deaths of hospital patients whose bodies are available for hospital autopsy}} \times 100$$

Fetal Death Rate

$$\frac{\text{Total number of intermediate and/or late fetal deaths for a period}}{\text{Total number of live births} + \text{intermediate and late fetal deaths for the period}} \times 100$$

Neonatal Mortality Rate (Death Rate)

$$\frac{\text{Total number of newborn deaths for a period}}{\text{Total number of newborn infant discharges (including deaths) for the period}} \times 100$$

Maternal Mortality Rate (Death Rate)

$$\frac{\text{Total number of direct maternal deaths for a period}}{\text{Total number of obstetrical discharges (including deaths) for the period}} \times 100$$

Caesarean-Section Rate

$$\frac{\text{Total number of caesarean sections performed in a period}}{\text{Total number of deliveries in the period (including caesarean sections)}} \times 100$$